The Fitness Director's Guide to Marketing Strategies & Tactics

by Richard F. Gerson, Ph.D.

ISBN No. 0-944183-14-X
Library of Congress No. 92-082570

Published by:
Professional Reports Corporation
4571 Stephen Circle, N.W.
Canton, Ohio 44718-3629

Cover design by:
Laurance C. Herbert

Distributed by:
Professional Reports Corporation
4571 Stephen Circle, N.W.
Canton, Ohio 44718-3629

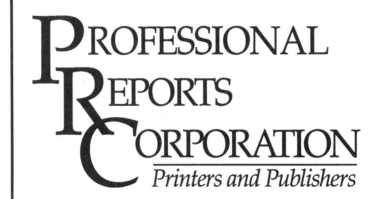

4571 Stephen Circle NW • Canton, Ohio 44718-3629
(216) 499-0205 • 1-800-336-0083 • FAX (216) 499-6609

Table of Contents

Dedication

This book is dedicated with much love and gratitude to my primary target market, my family: my wife, Robbie, and our two sons, Michael and Mitchell.

About The Author

Richard F. Gerson, Ph.D., CMC, CPC, is President of Gerson Goodson, Inc., a marketing and management consulting firm. Richard is also a nationally renowned speaker and trainer who has made presentations to tens of thousands of people at numerous corporations and at national and international meetings.

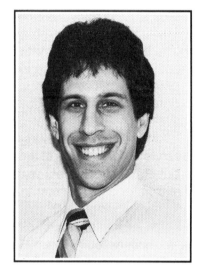

Dr. Gerson received his Ph.D. from Florida State University in 1978. He has consulted with both large and small businesses, including entrepreneurial start-ups as well as Fortune 500 companies. He has also worked with many professional membership organizations to enhance their marketing efforts.

Richard became a Certified Professional Consultant (CPC) in 1991 and a Certified Management Consultant in 1992. These certifications assure his clients of the utmost in professional ethics, service and quality performance.

Richard has published several books. Aside from this publication, his latest is **WRITING AND IMPLEMENTING A MARKETING PLAN** and **BEYOND CUSTOMER SERVICE**, published by Crisp Publications. He has also published over 200 articles on various topics in popular and professional magazines.

Richard's consulting philosophy has always focused on three things: 1) Work with each client exclusively in their area during the term of the agreement; 2) Provide superior customer service at all times, and; 3) Assist the client to become self sufficient and independent. These philosophies have been the key to Richard's success for over 14 years.

Preface

The fitness industry has become extremely competitive during the latter part of the 1980s and the early 1990s. There is also every indication that the industry will become even more competitive as more and more branches of fitness and related activities and programs vie for the same consumer dollar. Where once there were just exercise facilities and health clubs, now there are wellness centers, aerobics studios, personal training facilities, health promotion facilities, weight loss centers, diabetes management centers, cardiac rehabilitation programs, and the list goes on.

All these areas promote the concept of fitness, or wellness, as being integral to a healthy lifestyle. And directors of these programs all want the customer to come to them to purchase products and services. In fact, the high level of competition has caused many fitness directors and program managers to vertically and horizontally integrate their programs.

For example, health clubs that once were only weight lifting gyms or exercise studios now teach aerobics, offer stress management lectures, provide weight loss programs and products, give massages, and even bring in physicians to do medical evaluations. This integration of services is an attempt to keep the member/customer in one location and develop loyalty in that customer.

Every program in the country claims to have highly qualified and well trained individuals on their staff. Fitness directors also claim to all have the best program, the most effective program, the safest program, or the most results-oriented program. Now you and I both know that not everyone can have the best or be the best. There has to be some distinction, but you would never know it from the marketing messages these facilities send out. So, since everyone is the best and offers the best, how do you distinguish your program from your competitors?

The answer is simple. Develop a strategically based, tactically oriented marketing program. Make sure the foundation of the program is solid, based on facts and good strategies. Then, develop tactics to implement those strategies. For example, if your goal is to increase participation in a weight loss program, you should first target your current members, then communicate with the public. Your public marketing campaign should include some advertising, some public relations, as much free publicity as possible, and a specific message targeted to a specific group of people. You also must develop a tracking program to determine how effective your marketing program truly is.

That is the essence of effective marketing. You determine who you want to do business with you, find out what they need, want and expect, then you tell them and show them how you will give them all that and more. Then, you give it to them as you provide superior customer service to keep them as customers for life.

Richard F. Gerson, Ph.D.

What This Book Is About

This book is about marketing, in its entirety as it relates to the fitness industry. The fitness industry, for purposes of the book, includes wellness, health promotion, aerobics, personal training, weight loss, exercise and anything else that would use fitness as a criteria for a lifestyle change. The book is designed for fitness directors, wellness center directors, program managers, facility managers, supervisors, and anyone else in the fitness industry who needs to learn about marketing. Actually, I guess that means everybody.

Marketing is an umbrella term for all the activities you would use to communicate with your prospects and customers. This includes advertising, public relations, sales and sales promotions, charity events, community events, in-house programs, and anything else that requires getting a message out to the buying public. Marketing also includes research, planning, implementation and evaluation of the programs.

You will learn how to develop successful ads, write quality copy and press releases, sell your programs and services, and provide superior customer service. Go through the book slowly, identify the three to five strategies and tactics that you think will help you the most, and concentrate on making these work. It is always better to do a few things successfully than to do a lot of things poorly.

If you have any questions, or need help after going through the book, feel free to write me at the address below or call me.

Lastly, I must thank David Herbert and Professional Reports Corporation for publishing this book. Without their belief in the content and the importance of the topic, this book would never have been written. Thank you.

Richard F. Gerson, Ph.D.
Gerson Goodson, Inc.
P.O. Box 1534
Safety Harbor, Florida 34695
(813) 726-7619

Developing A Marketing Plan

Chapter 1

Planning for Success

The telephone call came very early in the morning. The voice at the other end of the line was frantic. It was an old friend whom I had not heard from for years. She was telling me she was in trouble. She had recently opened a commercial fitness center with all the latest high-tech equipment, qualified instructors, beautiful amenities, and high hopes. She had everything a member could want in a club. The only thing she did not have was members.

After I got her to calm down somewhat, I asked her what her plan was to succeed in this commercial fitness venture. "Plan?", she asked. "What plan? I just thought I could open a club, and since I had a large following as an instructor, all my students would come and join my club to help me get started. Unfortunately, it did not happen that way. In fact, the club is almost empty. Now, what am I supposed to do?"

It was quite obvious to me, although not to my friend, what the problem was. She had all the right elements for fitness club success except one. She did not plan how she was going to make her venture successful. And that planning requires a specific type of plan: a marketing plan, to be exact.

The Importance of Planning for Success

It is very important to plan for your success. Planning does not necessarily require a 5 or 10 year, long-term strategic plan, although you should plan for future events. Planning, at a minimum, requires you to determine exactly what you would like to do and probably will do within the next three, six and twelve months of your business.

The fitness field is changing rapidly, and your planning efforts must be flexible enough to adapt to the changing marketplace. This is especially true of your marketing plan. Planning for success in today's fitness marketplace requires flexibility and adaptability. You cannot be married to a plan or your planning process. You need to be able to change immediately when the marketplace changes, such as a new competitor moving in the area, or when your members' needs change.

The importance of planning cannot be emphasized enough. Remember, though, that in order to plan for your success, you must plan strategically to a point and tactically to operate and survive on a daily basis. Your marketing plan will help you do this.

The Purpose of a Marketing Plan

A marketing plan serves a very important purpose related to the success of your fitness venture, whether it is a commercial club, aerobics studio, personal training business, wellness center, cardiac rehabilitation center, or a health promotion program. Marketing is your key to success.

The primary purpose of a marketing plan is to act as your guide and roadmap as you operate your business. Fitness directors, whether they are employees or owners, tend to know a great deal about fitness and not enough about how to market their expertise. The marketing plan takes you step by step to inform the public about your expertise and why you are better for them than your competitors.

A good marketing plan is action-oriented. It is usable on a daily basis. The fitness director can refer to it to help him or her through a variety of situations. Each component of the marketing plan should describe how you would handle and succeed in a given situation. Marketing jargon and techno-speak have no place in today's rapidly changing fitness business environment. Therefore, when you develop and write your marketing plan, keep it short, simple, sweet and action-oriented.

Components of a Marketing Plan

Written marketing plans have a variety of subsections with different titles. However, most of the titles are just ease-of-use conventions for the authors. The components I am recommending to you here are fairly universal and very simple to work with. You can find a more extensive discussion of these components in my other marketing book for the fitness industry, **MARKETING HEALTH/FITNESS SERVICES**, published by Human Kinetics Publishers.

Every marketing plan must begin with a cover page followed by an Executive Summary. This is a brief description of the contents of the plan. The Executive Summary should be no more than two to four pages long and should give the reader enough information about the plan to determine if they want to go on reading the entire written document.

The next section of the marketing plan is the Target Market Analysis or the Market Segmentation procedures. Here you determine the people with whom you want to do business. You can also call this section a Customer Analysis.

Identify your customers or target market by as many characteristics as possible. For example, where do they live, how much money do they make, how will they pay for the fitness services and memberships, what is their level of education, where do they work, how much free time do they have, will they be paying for your services with needed income or discretionary funds, how high on their value hierarchy is your fitness membership, what needs, wants and expectations do they have of you and your facility, and what type of service do they require?

These are just some of the questions you need to answer to begin writing a marketing plan that will help you be successful. Notice that the questions cover the customer segmentation areas of demographics, geographics, psychographics and sociographics. There are also questions about their lifestyles and their customer service requirements.

Once you can answer all these questions completely, you are ready to determine how well you stack up in the marketplace. Now you can begin your in-depth market research into your competitors and to the deeper needs of the customers.

The Market Research section of the marketing plan will help you determine your marketing strategies and tactics, your promotional efforts, and anything else you will do to communicate your intentions to the buying public. If the health-conscious individual does not know why he or she should work out at your facility, or if you do not know how to reach them, then your market research has been faulty and your subsequent marketing communications will be faulty.

There are basically two types of market research: primary and secondary. Primary research is information and data you collect yourself through surveys, telephone interviews and personal meetings with customers. This is usually more time consuming and expensive than secondary research, but there are situations that require the precision of primary research.

Secondary research is your interpretation of information that has been previously collected for other situations. Many fitness directors use local newspapers, census data and Standard Industrial Codes (SIC) as sources of secondary data to find and classify their customers. You should identify the sources of secondary data that will be most helpful to you in writing your plan and successfully operating your fitness business.

Your market research must also include information about your competitors. There are many sources for this information. The first, and most accessible, is to ask your employees, or former employees of your competitors, about your competitors. They are usually very happy to tell you. Next, read the newspapers and trade magazines for information. Watch for their ads and press notices. Also, you can use the list on the next page to help you find more information about your competitors.

Competitor Information Sources

I. Competitor Sources
    A. Direct inquiry
    B. Facility visits/Direct observation
    C. Current or former employees of competitors
    D. Speeches
    E. Company publications and brochures
    F. Press releases and news stories
    G. Financial reports
    H. Investor/stock information
    I. Advertisements
    J. Help wanted ads

II. Trade Sources
    A. Trade shows
    B. Trade publications
    C. Trade associations
    D. Professional organizations and meetings

III. Third Party Sources
    A. Customers
    B. Suppliers/vendors
    C. Distributors
    D. Other competitors
    E. Journalists/media contacts
    F. Consultants, accountants, lawyers
    G. Unions
    H. Your employees
    I. Dun & Bradstreet ratings
    J. Other sources you can find

IV. Published Sources
    A. Magazines and journals
    B. Bibliographies
    C. Directories
    D. Electronic data bases
    E. Reference books/mentions in other books
    F. University sources

You should also conduct an analysis of your competitors' **S**trengths, **W**eaknesses, the **O**pportunities you see in their weaknesses, and the **T**hreats they pose to you. This **SWOT** analysis, although very simple, is extremely effective in identifying the who, what, when, where and why of your competition.

When you have completed gathering all your information on your competitors and your customers, you are ready to begin developing your marketing mix. The Marketing Mix section of the plan describes the strategies and tactics you will use to market your fitness facility or services. The marketing mix contains sections such as what your product or service is, how, when and where it is going to be delivered, who are the people delivering it, what is the price of the product or service, are there any political or legal ramifications to your fitness product or service, and the promotional techniques you will use to inform the public about your fitness facility or services.

The Promotional Mix section of the plan follows and it should be a stand-alone section. Here you describe your advertising program, your public relations program, direct selling efforts, telemarketing efforts, sales promotion events, media events, grand openings, and anything else you would do to promote yourself and/or your facility.

The next section of the plan details the results you expect to achieve. This is a check on the goals you should have written in the strategies and tactics section. Your marketing results can be in market share, dollars of annual revenue, number of members, or anything else you want to use to define your marketing results.

The last section of the plan contains all your documentation, such as sample ads you plan to use for the time period of the marketing plan, media scripts (commercials for radio and television), sample press releases, legal documents, contracts, and anything else that may have an effect on your marketing.

Writing the Plan

Now that you have collected all this information, you must write the marketing plan. First, decide on your time frame for the plan. You may want to write a one-year plan and then break it down into 90 day segments. Whatever time frame you choose, be sure to write the marketing plan in an action-oriented manner. Make it simple enough so that a ten year old can understand it. Keep the plan dynamic, flexible and alive. Use it on a daily basis. It is the only way you can guarantee your success.

Starting Business

Chapter 2

Open for Business

You are now ready to conduct your fitness business. It does not matter whether you are a full size commercial fitness center, a corporate program, an aerobics studio, a hospital-based center, a personal trainer, or any other type of fitness business. You have to let the world know you are open and ready for them. The way to do this is through a variety of marketing and public relations techniques.

We can assume at this point that you have all your licenses, identification numbers, permits and anything else you need to operate your fitness business in your chosen location. Now you must tell the public who you are, where you are, what you do, and how and why you do it better than anyone else.

Traditional Marketing Techniques

There are some traditional, tried and true marketing techniques that will work to get your name out in front of the public. You should follow these techniques because they work. If you want to adapt them, make sure your modification only improves them and you are not changing them just for personal ego gratification. These same techniques are used by the largest companies all over the world.

➤ Press Release

This is the most common technique. Simply write up a press release and send it to your local media. The release should contain information on your business, what you do, when you are opening, and the products and services you offer. This initial release is simply an announcement, not a sales presentation. You may want to include a picture of yourself and/or your facility with the release. Press releases with pictures tend to get printed more often and responded to more rapidly by radio and television media.

The following page shows you a sample format and content of a basic announcement release. I have used this approach hundreds of times for clients, both in and out of the fitness industry, and it has never failed yet. There is always some mention of the opening of the new business in one or more publications.

Change the words and the content to suit your specific needs. Remember that in this release and in any other release you will write, the material should be newsworthy and go from the specific to the general. The media may not have time to read your entire release so you must get them the most important information in the first paragraph or two. Also, if possible, keep all releases to one or two pages.

News Release

DATE: Current Date
CONTACT: Richard F. Gerson
TELEPHONE: (xxx) xxx-xxxx

FOR IMMEDIATE RELEASE

ULTIMATE FITNESS CENTER NOW OPEN

Safety Harbor, Florida -Richard Gerson announces the opening of the Ultimate Fitness Center located at 1234 USA St. in Safety Harbor, Florida. The Ultimate Fitness Center has state-of-the-art fitness equipment, a lap and exercise pool, a 2500 square foot aerobics room, separate free weight rooms and locker rooms for men and women, certified fitness professionals, and licensed massage therapists, physical therapists and cosmetologists. The center also offers members an Alpha Workout, which is a 30 minute private session in a relaxation room designed to help you manage your stress.

The Ultimate Fitness Center is open 7 days a week from 6:00 am to 10:00 pm. Memberships are available on an individual and family basis. Special memberships are also available for children, students and seniors. Babysitting is free.

For more information, call (xxx) xxx-xxxx.

#

Notice several things about this press release. The important information is right at the beginning. You can go even further and describe the "state-of-the-art" equipment, which would make the facility even more impressive. Also, there is a second mention of the telephone number to call. You want to make sure that those who receive your press release as well as those who will read it in a newspaper know how to get in touch with you. Finally, you end the release with the symbol "###" or "-30-". These are basic conventions that are used in the industry.

Follow the same formula for all your press releases. Put yourself on a schedule to send out a release every month, every quarter or every six months. They key is to keep your name and your business in front of the media and the public. Just remember that the press release must have something newsworthy in it or the recipients will start to file them in the garbage as soon as they receive them.

Press releases are one of the least expensive marketing techniques you can use, and they are often one of the most effective. For the price of paper and a postage stamp, you have the possibility of receiving what amounts to free advertising in newspapers, on radio or on television.

Now, don't limit your marketing to just your local area. If you want to create a national image and reputation, send your releases to trade magazines, professional associations and trade newsletters. Also, put other people in the fitness industry on your mailing list. You never know who will receive a press release and pass it along to someone else who may want to do business with you.

➤ The Press Release Article

Media people receive many press releases from all types of industries. Sometimes, they are inundated with them and they don't even read them. Therefore, you must make your release stand out from the crowd. One way is to make it look innovative and attractive to the reader.

I use something I call the press release article. It is a press release written in a two column format to resemble a newspaper article. It also has a heading on it like a newspaper article. The heading can be straight black print on white paper or it can be reversed out. The choice is yours.

The reason for using the press release article instead of the traditional press release is two-fold. First, it stands out simply by the fact that the format is different. Most people do not send press releases with bold, glaring headlines to capture the reader's attention. When you do this, your information about your fitness business stands out.

The second reason is that a press release in article format has a good chance of getting printed as an article by a newspaper. They do not have to rewrite it nor do they have to re-format it. They simply have to typeset it and print it. So, if you are a good writer, put your skills to work and send your press releases in article format. Again, keep the length to one or two pages.

The following sample shows you exactly what this type of press release looks like. When you send these to newsletter publishers, they tend to publish them because the article is already written.

NEW BOOK TEACHES FITNESS DIRECTORS HOW TO MARKET THEIR BUSINESSES EFFECTIVELY AND INEXPENSIVELY

Safety Harbor, Florida – Richard F. Gerson, Ph.D., has recently published a new book for the fitness industry entitled **THE FITNESS DIRECTOR'S GUIDE TO MARKETING STRATEGIES AND TACTICS**. The book is published by Professional Reports Corporation.

The fitness industry has some of the most technically competent professionals in any industry in the world, said Dr. Gerson. Many of these expert technicians lack the knowledge or experience in marketing that is necessary to compete successfully in the business world. That is the reason for the book.

The guide is a comprehensive and practical manual on how to develop marketing programs and implement them for all aspects of the fitness industry. The reader is provided information on how to write a marketing plan, how to conduct market research, how to advertise and promote their fitness business, how to develop and get free publicity, and how to use customer service as a marketing tool.

The book also provides over 130 low cost or no cost marketing techniques for fitness directors to use when marketing their business. Some of these techniques are tried and true while others are very

novel and unique. All of them have been used by Dr. Gerson in the past and have met with success.

Also included in the book are over 50 suggestions on how to establish a customer service and member retention program, and then how to use these as marketing tools. Additionally, there are charts and forms for readers to use to develop their own marketing programs.

This is the eighth book by Dr. Gerson and the second on marketing for the fitness industry. He has also recently published **BEYOND CUSTOMER SERVICE** and is currently writing another book called **MEASURING QUALITY AND CUSTOMER SATISFACTION**.

Dr. Gerson is nationally known as a marketing consultant, and a corporate trainer in the areas of sales and marketing, customer service, quality improvement and communication skills. He has presented programs in all these areas at various conventions and meetings for fitness professionals and other organizations.

Dr. Gerson can be reached at (813) 726-7619 or P.O. Box 1534, Safety Harbor, Florida 34695.

➤ Backgrounders

Sometimes, you just cannot tell your fitness story in a traditional press release or the article format. You have too much to say to the public. You are bursting with information that you know they must have. In this case, you write a backgrounder to supplement the press release.

Use either format for the press release, then write an extensive background piece detailing everything you want your reader to know about your fitness business. There is no specified or required length for the backgrounder. There is also no particular format that you must follow, except that you should put a title on the piece, date it, and clearly write that it is a backgrounder.

The purpose of the backgrounder is to make certain you cover all the information you feel must be covered in order to give the reader a complete and clear picture of your business or your achievement. The media person reading the release and the backgrounder will determine what he or she finds interesting and usable. You are better off being comprehensive and letting them edit your backgrounder or call you to discuss it than being weak with the information.

Developing Your Media List

DON'T BUY A MEDIA LIST!! I must emphasize this strongly. New business owners, whether they are fitness professionals or in other fields, tend to want the quickest route to contacting the media. This is not the way to do it. First of all, the media list you buy or rent can be outdated. Second of all, you never know if it is correct. And, third, you are missing a great marketing opportunity when you buy a media list rather than build and develop your own.

Developing a media list is very simple, although it can be tedious. It is also a great marketing and public relations opportunity for you. Build your media list by doing the following.

Open your Yellow Pages to the sections on newspapers, radio stations, television stations and associations or organizations. Copy down each business name, address and telephone number. This will be much easier if you have a computer and a database program, but it can still be done by hand.

Once you have copied down all the pertinent information, call each business (newspaper, radio and television station, etc.), introduce yourself and your business, and ask who receives press releases. When you get the name, great. If they connect you to that person, even better. Introduce yourself and your business again, and ask that person when they like to receive press releases. Also, ask what in the fitness industry would impress them.

Sometimes, media companies have specific people who work in particular industries. If your local newspapers, radio or TV stations have someone who specializes in fitness, contact them, introduce yourself and ask the appropriate questions. Then, send them your press releases at the times they like to receive them. These times will usually coincide with their deadlines or in-between deadlines so they will have the chance to review your materials.

Many newspapers publish calendars of events. This information often must be sent to a specific person at a specific time, usually two weeks before the event. Get to know this person so that when you are hosting something at your fitness facility or doing something for the general public, they will look at your release first. Calendars of events publish information on a space available basis, and it is often first in, first printed.

OK. Now you have begun to develop your media list. You have canvassed the telephone books, made your calls and introductions, started your database, and now you are ready to send out releases. Wait! Your list is not complete.

Some of your best publicity will come from "little" newspapers, those that land on your driveway for free once a week or once a month. Get to know the editors and publishers of these papers and send them releases at the same time you send to the major players. Smaller, local papers, and even radio stations and cable television, are hungry for news, especially about local residents. Give them what they want on a regular basis, keep them on your media list, and they will repay you with more publicity and coverage than you could imagine or ever afford to pay for.

Your media list is still not complete, but you have developed a very usable list. Keep adding to the list, especially the names of trade and professional magazines and newsletters. Keep the list current, and if it is on your computer, make sure it is backed up on a disk. This could be one of your most important marketing possessions.

Invest in the paper and stamp to keep these people informed. You may even want to send releases to national magazines that are consumer oriented and that publish information on health and fitness. All you need is a mention in one of these magazines and you are instantly perceived as an expert. Think what this does for your image.

Building Your Professional Image

When it comes right down to it, your fitness business is really no different from your competitors down the street. Therefore, you must be able to differentiate yourself from them and in the minds of the consumers. These next several techniques will help you succeed where even large corporations fail. Don't be fooled by the fact that these marketing tactics are either low cost or no cost. The important thing to remember is that they work.

Businesses are made or broken by their images. This is more true for the fitness industry than anywhere else. You need both a physical appearance image and a professional business image. If one of these is lacking, your business can easily fail. Therefore, if you agree to continue working on your physical image, the following techniques will make you successful with your professional image.

Shaking Hands, Patting Backs and Kissing Babies

Get out and meet people. Introduce yourself and your business. Ask them to tell you about what they do, and then tell them about what you do. The more people you meet, the more opportunities you have to market your business. And remember, if someone you meet does not join your facility or become a client, they can always refer you to someone else. Therefore, view everyone you meet as a potential client/member and treat them with the highest respect.

Be a Joiner

Several years ago I had a client who was a personal fitness trainer. This person had everything going for him. He was educated, certified, well built, attractive, communicative, and his business was going nowhere fast. The problem was very simple. This trainer knew he had all these positive attributes so he felt they elevated him above the crowd and the competition. Therefore, clients would and should come to him. Right? Wrong!

I had this personal trainer join a local chamber of commerce, become involved with a charity, join two local professional organizations, and agree to speak to local business and professional groups on a variety of fitness topics for free. Business went from one client to 23 inside of three months. Now, the trainer has two other trainers working for him, and they are members of organizations.

No matter what you think of local chambers of commerce or professional organizations, no matter how many people have told you that they never received one client from their memberships in these organizations, no matter how many people tell you it is a waste of your money, I am telling you now to "waste" your money. JOIN your local chamber and at least two professional organizations. Attend the meetings and offer to work on committees. Volunteer for a charity.

You may not receive business in the short term, but down the road people will start to refer clients and members to you. People and companies have different motivations to buy fitness services, and they have different buying cycles. You can assure yourself of being there for them when they are ready by being a member and participating with them. Also, offer to speak at their meetings, even if it is for free. The more they get to know you, the more they will like you, and the more they will eventually want to do business with you.

5 Ways to Create an Expert Image

➤ Creating Expertise: Part 1

Much of your image is based on how you are perceived by the public. If you are perceived as the expert in health and fitness, then people will look to you for advice and come to you to do business. Here is the first way to create that image of an expert.

Get certified, then send out a press release announcing that you have received this national, professional certification. This certification signifies that you have an extensive body of knowledge in your field and that you provide high quality service while maintaining the clients' best interests. Send out a press release each time you receive a new certification. People love initials and credentials. They will look to you as an expert.

➤ Creating Expertise: Part 2

Call and write your local media contacts and inform them that you are available as a local resource for any questions they may have in the health and fitness field. Any time there is something in the news about fitness, such as a new discovery or recommendation for exercise, write or call these contacts and offer your opinion. Eventually, someone will ask you to give your name and business. Once you are mentioned in print or on radio or television, you are perceived by the public as an expert. So, become a resource for the media.

➤ Creating Expertise: Part 3

Write and publish. It does not matter where you publish, just publish. Call your local, small newspapers and ask them if they want a column on fitness. Write it for free. All you want is the byline and the ability to clip the article and use it as a publicity piece.

If no one will let you write for them, publish your own material. Write a pamphlet on training techniques, for example, and send a press release to the papers saying the pamphlet is available for free. When people respond, send it to them with your business card. People believe what they read in print. Since your name is on the published document, you must be an expert.

Take this a step further and publish your own book, magazine or newsletter. It does not matter what it is, as long as it is a published work. Then use the publication as a publicity piece to promote your business.

If you think it is difficult to publish your own book, think again. Several years ago, I was asked to present a marketing workshop for an international fitness director's organization. No one, in any professional fitness organization, had ever presented a three hour marketing program before this one. Obviously, the turnout was going to be great, and it was even better than expected. So, knowing I had a captive audience, I took everything one step further and wrote a training manual on marketing fitness services. This was sold at the workshop and 85 people paid $20 each for that manual.

This gave me instant credibility as a marketing expert in the fitness field. What was even better was that a year later, a major trade publishing house requested that I revise the manual and they would publish it as a hard cover book. The revisions were made and the first marketing book for the health/fitness industry was published in 1989.

Here is one other story. A former client of mine mentioned that he had written a manuscript that he felt made a contribution to the fitness field. However, he did not have anyone to publish it. I recommended he publish it himself, sell it at conferences and workshops, and then shop it around for a publisher. Once a publisher sees you have a track record of selling your book, they are more inclined to take a chance on publishing your first book.

He followed my advice and in 1991, published his first book with a national publishing house. I know that when I received my copy of the book I was almost as proud of him as he was of himself. Now, he is positioned as an expert in his area of the fitness industry, which is fitness management and programming.

I tell you these stories to encourage you to write and publish your own material. You never know where it may lead, but you can be certain that it will always enhance your credibility and your image as an expert in your field. Why do you think you are reading this book now? Because it adds to my credibility and my image as a marketing consultant in the fitness industry. Again, I encourage you to write and publish.

➤ Creating Expertise: Part 4

Speak. Call all the local organizations you can find, ask to speak to their program director, and then offer your services as a speaker at one of their meetings. Everyone is interested in some aspect of health and fitness, so you have a built-in audience. You just have to be able to get on their program.

Many people ask me about charging a fee for their speaking. I recommend the following. If you are just starting out, never charge. You should be thrilled that other professionals want to hear what you have to say. Once you have established a track record, then you can begin asking the organizations if they pay a speaker's honorarium. If they do, accept what they offer. If they don't, speak anyway as you should not pass up the opportunity to meet new people.

After you have become recognized as an expert and a "professional" speaker, then you can start setting your own fees. Remember not to price yourself out of an engagement by being to costly. The more people who hear you speak, the more speeches you will be offered, and the more potential clients/members you will have.

➤ Creating Expertise: Part 5

Experts advise, so get on an advisory board. This can be an advisory board to a company, a charity, or a civic organization. When people hear you are on an advisory board, they will instantly have respect for your expertise and want to do business with you rather than your competitors.

Be careful, though. Membership on advisory boards can become addicting, so don't overextend yourself. If you are asked to sit on more than one board, you must choose those boards whom you can best serve and who will provide you with the greatest potential for increasing your business. If you spread yourself too thin, your "expertise" will start to deteriorate and your professional image will suffer.

Don't Forget These Important Image Builders

Look at your business card. Do you like it? Does it portray the image you want it to portray? Does it send the message you intended it to send? If not, or if you are not sure, then change your business card.

The business card is one of the least expensive and most important marketing tools you can use. Never skimp on a business card. Make certain it has all the pertinent information such as company name, address, telephone and fax numbers, your name, and anything else you think must be on it without cluttering it up. If you do not have artistic or creative ability, it is wise to pay an artist to design a logo and business card for you.

Have the card printed on quality stock, and if you need color to express your message, use it. Also, you may want to consider a photo business card. This approach can show a picture of you working out, with a client, or of your facility. Photo business cards are obviously very eye catching, but they do have one drawback. Sometimes, it is difficult to print over the color photo. Check with your local printer or supplier of these types of cards before you invest. They do cost more than regular business cards.

The reason business cards are so important is because people expect you to have them and use them. The easiest way to give someone a business card is to ask them for theirs first. They will politely respond in kind or graciously accept yours as you offer it to them. You may even want to give them two cards, one for a friend (see "Referral").

Along with your business card goes your letterhead. Keep the logos and print styles similar, and the quality of the letterhead must be equal to that of the business cards. Have your envelopes match your letterhead in content and quality, although it is not necessary to reprint your logo on the envelopes if it is on the letterhead.

This advice may seem very simplistic, but you would be surprised how many business professionals, both in the fitness industry and outside, do not pay enough attention to their business cards, letterhead and envelopes.

Looking the Part

Now you have some basic advice on how to create your expert image. Later in the book we will discuss how to develop professional literature such as brochures and flyers. For now, you have to create the packaging that goes along with your business, and that packaging is you.

If you are going to act the part of the fitness professional, you must look and live the part. You must be in shape, both physically and mentally. Your appearance is your packaging. You would not want to work out with someone who was fat and slovenly, or looked weak and tired. Why should you expect someone else to do the same just for you?

Live the lifestyle you are professing to be an expert in. Let everyone see how healthy and fit you are. When it comes right down to it, all your brochures and literature may not make the sale, no matter how well done they are, if you do not look and act like a fitness professional.

Another important aspect of looking the part is matching your appearance to the client whom you are trying to secure or work with. For example, if you are trying to sell a major corporation on your fitness programs, and you have an appointment with the president, it is probably a good idea to go to that appointment dressed professionally rather than in a workout outfit. Let the prospect see that you, too, are a business professional, and you treat your business and your clients with the same respect that other businesses do theirs.

On the other hand, if you are approaching a country club and the contact person tells you to come casual, make certain you dress in that manner. The more you can match your appearance to that of your clients and prospects, the better your chances are of securing more business. Plus, your clients will now market for you because they like you and perceive that you are like them. Do you know of a better marketing technique than referrals and word of mouth?

Word of Mouth Advertising

Chapter 3

A Primer On Word-Of-Mouth Marketing

Eavesdrop with me on a conversation between two friends over lunch. One has just come from working out at a local health club and is telling the other about the club. The second friend was considering joining the club. Here is the conversation.

"That was probably the worst workout I ever had. The aerobics instructor was late, and when I went to work on the CV equipment, it was broken. I asked someone when it would be fixed and they did not know. There wasn't even a sign on the equipment letting members know it was out of order. Plus, the locker room smells like it hasn't been cleaned for weeks and the seats on the weight equipment are all torn up. Even though I have six months left on my membership, I don't know if I am going back there."

"You know, I was thinking about joining your club, but after what you are saying, I probably will have to look somewhere else. I certainly don't want to be in a club that has broken equipment, instructors who don't care, and staff members who don't know what is going on. Thanks for helping me make my decision."

Now I know this is a very negative conversation, and to be truthful, there are many positive conversations between friends that get people to join clubs. The purpose of telling you a negative story is to impress upon you how powerful negative word of mouth marketing can be. In fact, it can be four to five times more powerful than positive word of mouth. Therefore, you have to do everything within your control to develop a positive word-of-mouth marketing program.

Developing a Word-of-Mouth Marketing Program

People from all fields of business are under the misconception that they cannot control a word-of-mouth marketing program. That is absolutely not true. You have already learned in the previous chapter some of the things you can do to positively affect word-of-mouth. Speeches, publications, committees and other credibility builders will help spread the word about your fitness business. What you need to do is control this talk factor in a planned and prescribed manner, as much as possible.

Your word-of-mouth marketing program begins with what you are selling, either a fitness product or service. Make sure this is a quality product or service and has a high perceived value by the customer. Otherwise, you will have difficulty generating positive word-of-mouth. Once you have your product or service, decide on the message you want to send about it. This message must tell the public all the benefits they will receive from working out with you. Then, you must get the message to the people.

The first way to get the message out is to listen to what is coming in. Listen to your current members or clients and your employees. What are they saying about you and your business? Is it good or bad? Are there things you should be paying more attention to? What can you do to improve on what they are saying?

Check your records to see how many new members are the result of referrals from current clients? If your membership or client base is not at least 80% referrals by your third year, then what are you doing that is not attracting this business? Also, why do people refer to you while others do not? What are the reasons new members have for joining your facility or becoming your clients? Pay strict attention to the communications that go on among members, employees, and members and employees. This invaluable information about your business and its chances for continued growth and success will help you determine the effectiveness of your overall marketing program. Once you know what people are saying about you, you can begin to manage your word-of-mouth marketing program.

Where To Begin

Begin your word-of-mouth marketing program internally with your employees. If you are a sole practitioner, then begin with yourself and program yourself for positive comments and attitudes about your business. Work with and train your employees so that they know more than just their job. They should know everything about the fitness business, inside and outside. Share all your knowledge and information with them, even what was once considered proprietary information. The more your employees know about the business, the more they can do to promote it.

Show your employees that you live the mission of your fitness business. Let them see and experience your positive attitude so that they, in turn, can develop the same type of attitude and commitment. Train them, nurture them and reward them for their behaviors. Teach them what to say to whom and when to say it. Then, let them instill their own personalities into their jobs and empower them to make decisions to help the members. These few behaviors on your part will motivate employees to have the proper attitude about your fitness business and to go out and promote it to the community.

It is important to have all your employees speaking positively about the fitness business. You will also find that one or two employees really stand out above the rest. They are your "champions". Work with them to make them even more of your "marketing mouthpieces" to get the word out. Have them speak before community and professional groups and sit on committees. Make them an integral part of your business and marketing and you will be rewarded with a successful fitness business.

One other note about beginning your word-of-mouth marketing program internally. Your employees are also your customers. We will discuss later in this book about the importance of customer service and how and why you must treat your employees as customers. For now, understand that the success of your word-of-mouth marketing program also depends on the quality of the customer service you provide to your employees.

The Next Step

Your next step in controlling the word-of-mouth marketing program is to work with your members. Take a lesson from the very popular step workout and start small and work up to more difficult heights and routines.

Begin by being visible to your customers and talking with them on a regular basis. Get their opinions and suggestions on how you can make things better for them on a regular basis. Ask them why they do business with you, why they decided to join your facility instead of someone else's. Ask them why they stay with you instead of changing clubs, trainers or instructors. Once you have asked these questions, listen very carefully to the answers.

If you just listen to them, you will have more information about your own business and your competitors' businesses than you ever dreamed possible. You will be able to structure your entire marketing program to take advantage of the many opportunities your customers present to you. The more you listen to them, the more of them will go out and market for you. When you start to implement their suggestions internally, your external "sales" force multiplies exponentially.

Help your members market for you. Give them simple yet effective things to tell their friends. Remember the step workout. After they have become a referral source for you, cultivate them and give them even more information to tell their friends. The more you get them involved in your fitness business, the more involved they will want to become and remain.

Remember, you need to train your customers to provide referrals for you. Referrals will just not come because you do a good job or you happen to be a nice person. You must first train them in what types of referrals you want, then ask them for the referrals, and then help them make the referrals to you.

As customers make referrals to your fitness business, you must develop a reward program to thank them. We will discuss some of these ideas later in the book. For now, think of how you want to recognize and reward the positive word-of-mouth that your customers and members are generating for you.

Other Ways to Generate Positive Word of Mouth

As the chapter subtitle stated, this is just a primer on how to develop a word-of-mouth marketing program. While books have been written on the subject, you will be successful if you just do the things mentioned here. Now, here are several other ways for you to generate positive word-of-mouth.

Be novel. Be outrageous or outlandish. Be unique. Be different. Do something different. Host an extra special, special event. And always, make sure whatever you do is positive and has a good and beneficial outcome for everyone.

People love novelty and uniqueness. In fact, there was something unique about you that made them become your customer in the first place. Now, do something else new and unique. Keep your fitness business fresh. Ask people for new ideas and try them out. And contact the media. If it's new, they may want to cover it. Once they cover it, you have tremendous word-of-mouth about your fitness business.

So that's it. Your basic primer on word-of-mouth marketing. Start with your employees, work with your customers, and recognize and reward everyone for their efforts. Be unique and different, and keep the media informed of newsworthy events occurring in your fitness business. Use word-of-mouth to generate publicity for your business and then be prepared to benefit from the publicity.

One Last Thought

There is a publicity-generating technique that some people include as part of their word-of-mouth marketing program. It is called "seeding". Seeding is when you or someone else calls up the media, or any other influential person, as someone other than yourself, and requests information on your fitness business. You are "planting a seed" in their minds about some feature of your business. When enough people do this, the media person begins to think there may be a story behind this fitness business. They may call you and do that story, which does generate the publicity you were seeking. However, be aware of two things.

First, if they find there is really no story there, what can their negative word-of-mouth do to your business? You can't fight city hall nor can you fight the media. Similarly, along those same lines, what happens to you if this influential person finds out you were seeding the story? How will you deal with their thoughts, feelings and negative word-of-mouth?

Many companies, both large and small, seed their publicity stories to generate the word-of-mouth they desire. I am not saying it is good or bad. I am presenting it to you as another technique for your word-of-mouth marketing program. You must decide if and when and how you are going to use it.

You must also remember that word-of-mouth marketing is not a substitute for a good marketing plan and an overall marketing program. Word-of-mouth is just one component of a comprehensive marketing plan, and like other aspects of that plan, it must be controlled and used to achieve its desired benefits.

You should never leave your word-of-mouth marketing to chance. Use the techniques mentioned here and make word of mouth work for you. You will find it a positive addition to your marketing program.

Direct Response Advertising

Chapter 4

Marketing Through Direct Response

I recently received a call from a fitness director who did not understand why her marketing program and advertising campaigns were not working. Her facility was spending over $1,000 a week in newspaper ads, flyers and mailers, and these materials were not generating the desired number of responses. Since this is a great deal of money to be spending without receiving an appropriate return, I fully understood why she was upset. I asked her to send me her materials so that I could review them. Here is what I found.

The newspaper ads were of the copycat, everyday variety that said get in shape for XXX amount of dollars. There was a telephone number and the address of the facility, but they were in small print. The flyers were simple, one page descriptions of memberships with the club name and phone number on them. Nothing fancy or eye catching. Finally, the direct mail pieces were just brochures about the club. The suggestions I gave her will help you improve your direct marketing campaigns, so please follow the advice closely.

The Basics of Direct Response Marketing

First and foremost, **ALL** marketing **MUST** be direct response. Informational marketing (or advertising), also known as institutional ads, are not very effective. They are more often a waste of money than a revenue generator. Your marketing must have a "call to action" in it. Something in your communication must motivate the reader to act now and become a customer/member.

For example, if you placed a newspaper ad and simply said **CALL NOW** with the telephone number in bigger, bolder letters than the rest of the ad, that is more effective than just giving the phone number. Your goal here is to increase the sense of urgency and time pressure for the reader to respond. Beef up your call now command with termination dates for the offer, like "expires on the 30th of this month," or "this offer is good only to the first 50 people who call". You must do something to generate a response.

Think of what motivates you to action. Ask your members what motivated them to join your facility or program. Ask people in the street what motivates them to exercise, and what de-motivates them. Gather as much practical information as possible and then use it as your call to action.

Remember that people like to be given direction and told how to do something, as well as what to do. When you place a newspaper ad that just gives information and does not tell the reader to call your club, you are wasting money. If you do not tell the reader to come in to tour the facility, or to join now before the membership rates increase, you are wasting money on that ad and marketing program

So, what did we do to improve the club's ad? We merely changed two things in the ad. *(Advertising techniques will be discussed later in the book. One aspect of successful advertising is mentioned here to help clarify the approach we took for the client and to emphasize how the entire ad works toward a direct response.)* We made the headline a benefit statement for the reader instead of an informational title. We also targeted the headline to a specific age group, which was 30 to 45 years old. We know from research that this age group does not want to grow old, gracefully or otherwise. They will fight it every "inch" of the way (weigh). We used this to create the benefit headline "If You Are Approaching Middle Age, You Do Not Have To Age In The Middle" and we showed pictures of people in this age group slightly out of shape with bulging middles as the before picture along with the same people in better shape as the after picture. This gets their interest.

The rest of the ad supported the headline and discussed some of the programs at the club. The call to action was to come in for a free workout or call to schedule a free personal training session. The idea here is to get people into the facility and then use the staff, facility and programs to sell them on a membership.

This change in the ad increased responses by over 200% and 30 new memberships were sold in one month, in addition to their average monthly sales.

There are several other simple to use, yet effective ways to increase response to a marketing communication. One of the best is a coupon. The coupon can be sent in for more information, to be placed in a prize pool, or to receive a discount on something. Lead boxes, which many commercial fitness centers use, are nothing more than information-requesting or prize-entering coupons.

We improved the club's flyers simply by adding a coupon at the bottom that required the customer to fill it in, mail it or bring it in for a free information brochure on how to start your own exercise program. While this may seem contradictory, since why would a club want someone to exercise at home instead of joining the facility, it really is not. In fact, the perception on the part of the customer is that if the club is willing to send me information on exercising at home, then the club must really have something great to offer for them to be so confident. Of course, the brochure emphasized using a home workout as a complement to a supervised club workout.

Another benefit of having people mail in the coupon is that the facility was now able to develop a mailing list of interested *(see Qualified)* prospects. These people could be contacted again and invited into the facility for a tour, a free trial membership, or anything else, and then sold a membership.

With respect to the mailers the club was using, brochures alone are never enough. We will go into more detail on direct mail procedures shortly, but you must realize that a letter always gets a better response than an information piece. A letter plus a brochure can also lead to an even greater response. Therefore, we just asked my friend to write a personal letter to the recipient inviting them to come to the club and ask for her personally. This improved the results of the direct mail campaign dramatically.

Summary of Direct Marketing Basics

Hopefully, at this point, you have learned a very inexpensive lesson compared to my friend described in the above story about how to successfully market your fitness programs. First, you make sure all your marketing communications, messages, advertising, and whatever, are direct response oriented. Use hidden commands such as call now, call this number, write, come in, or anything else that moves and motivates the person reading or hearing your message to do something about it. Also, use coupons to involve people in your marketing and to help you create a mailing list of interested prospects.

Second, if you use direct mail, always use an updated list and include a letter with your material. You must make sure your direct mail piece is delivered, and a good list increases your chances of reaching your prospective clients. Then, once you get the recipient to open the mail, they must read it. Letters are more personal and they tend to be read before they are thrown away. Letters are definitely read more often than information pieces. So, use a letter, even if you make the offer in the letter and send nothing else.

Third, you must be prepared to respond effectively to your direct marketing efforts. Make certain there are enough materials to send out in response to requests for information, there are enough staff members to tour potential members around the club and to provide them with the service and supervision they need during their free, trial workouts, and be available yourself to meet as many of these potential members as possible. When the fitness director pays personal attention to a prospective member, that person feels much more important and is more likely to join your program.

The Magic of Direct Mail: How to Make Clients and Members Appear Out of Thin Air

Somebody once said that direct mail can be the most expensive form of marketing because you never know if it is going to be successful and provide you with a return on your investment. That statement may be true, but it is usually true if your direct mail program does not follow the guidelines listed below. Someone else also said that a good response to a direct mail campaign is between 1% and 2%. Again, that may be true for some campaigns, but probably not if you follow these guidelines.

The first thing you do is make certain that direct mail fits in well with the rest of your marketing plan. If direct mail is just something you want to try because competitors are doing it, or it seems like a good idea, **STOP**. You will most certainly be wasting money.

Develop your direct mail programs as integral parts of your overall marketing plan. Then, when the timing is appropriate, roll out your direct mail campaign. Start with a small test area, and then if the materials and offer work, expand your market area. Never, never try a first-time direct mail campaign with a large market area.

7 Principles of Successful Direct Mail

Principle #1: Scratch the Niche

Many people think that the foundation of success in direct mail is the mailing list. The list is extremely important, as we will soon see. However, it is more important to first determine your target market. Who are the people you want to contact? What are their identifying characteristics? Basically, you are asking what niche market do they fit into.

I am a big proponent of two types of marketing, and neither includes being a small fish in a big pond. Many clubs opt for this approach because they figure there is enough to go around for everybody. I think they are wrong. You should either be a big fish in a little pond, or build your own pond (create your own niche market for your club). Then, you own the entire property (market).

After identifying your target market, you are ready to select your mailing list.

Principle #2: The Name's the Thing

Your mailing list will make or break your direct mail campaign. You must select your list carefully, and make sure it is current and accurate. There are two types of lists you can use: internal and external.

An internal mailing list comes from former members of your club and visitors. If you are not tracking everyone who comes into your facility and getting their name, address and telephone number, you should be because you are missing out on some tremendous money-making opportunities. Remember that these people have already shown an interest in what you are offering and they may just need a little of your positive motivation to get them to join. Keep this internal list up to date and ready for use.

Another way to generate an internal mailing list is to ask your employees and current members to provide you with three names and addresses whom they think might be interested in receiving information about the program. You will be surprised how many names you will get for your list just by asking. People want to help you succeed if you will just let them.

Your external mailing list will be much broader than your internal one. You must specify the characteristics of the people you want to reach. For example, specify their ages, gender, household income, residential or business zip code, number of family members, education level, purchasing habits, and anything else you can think of that will more narrowly define your potential prospects. When you have compiled all this information, you can either contact a list broker to rent or purchase a list for you, rent or purchase the list for yourself from other list owners, or you can look up names in the telephone book.

If you use a list broker, make certain the company can provide you with referrals and guarantees that the list is current and has been updated within the last three to six months. Also, make sure they will reimburse you in some way for non-deliverables — those pieces that are returned to you or trashed. You want to receive a guarantee that the list is at least 90% deliverable, or some other arrangement must be made, such as a reduction in price.

You can find list brokers in your telephone book under "mailing lists" or you can go to the library and read **DIRECT MAIL LISTS RATES AND DATA**, published by Standard Rate and Data Service.

Principle #3: Pay for Quality

Many fitness directors begin their first venture into direct mail by looking for the least expensive list that comes closest to meeting their specifications. This may work some of the time, but more often than not, you will find that you response is poor. As with anything else, **pay for quality**.

Lists usually cost between $10 and over $100 per thousand names. While the cost is important, it is only important in the context of how many of those names on the list have purchased fitness products or memberships, or how many of them have a predisposition to buy such items. The cost of a list does not determine its quality, although the more expensive lists usually contain names of the best mail order buyers and responders. Consider these lists when you decide on your campaign.

Depending on the number of names you want on a list, you may have to pay a premium. Or, the list owner or broker will tell you that you must purchase a minimum. If this is the case, purchase the minimum for your test market, test the list with your offer, and then buy more names to do a bigger mailing.

One more point about lists. You can purchase them on magnetic tape, which is usually done for extraordinarily large mailings, computer disks, or pressure labels. The price of the list may be affected by its format. Check this out carefully.

Principle #4: Make Them An Offer They Can't Refuse

Now you are ready to create your direct mail piece. Whatever you want to send to people, it must include an offer they cannot refuse. Your mail piece has to be so inviting and so motivating that they just have to call you or come see you now.

You can be as creative and artistic as you want, just don't get caught up in your own talent for creating this piece. Remember, it is still a sales tool, and as such, it must get the message across that the recipient will benefit more from joining your club than you will from having them there.

You are selling benefits, and benefits only. Forget features. People may be interested, albeit slightly, about the types of equipment or programs you may have. They are more interested in what these programs will do for them. They are not buying a membership. They are buying ways to realize their dreams, goals and hopes. Your club, facility or programs are just the vehicles for making that happen. Make sure your offer gives them exactly what they are hoping for and dreaming about.

For example, let's assume you decide that your direct mail campaign for your New Year's membership drive would focus around losing weight. You prepare your pieces for the mailing and wrap everything around a headline that says "Lose weight for the new year for only $19.92 a month". This headline will be ineffective for two reasons. The first is that most of your competitors are doing similar things and the second is that you have not communicated to the reader exactly what he or she really wants.

You know from your experience that losing weight is not the hard part. The difficulty comes in keeping the weight off. Your headline should communicate this benefit of how your program makes losing weight easy and keeping it off even easier. Once this captures your readers' attention, you can be sure they will read everything else. Then, since your offer is so motivating, they will call you for an appointment.

Principle #5: Check Your Calendar

Never do a direct mail program indiscriminately. You should know from research in the fitness industry what the peak buying months are. Schedule your mailing to coincide with those peak buying months. For example, most people join clubs during January to lose weight and stick to their New Year's Resolutions. Your offer should focus on how you will help them achieve this and the mailing should arrive after Christmas.

Let me give you an example from a personal trainer I worked with in South Florida. This person wanted to do a direct mail program to secure new clients and followed most of the above advice. However, the timing of the mailing was bad. The offer was to get in shape for summer at a discounted price. I suggested mailing the piece in April for a discounted workout series in May, since people perceive that summer is June, July and August. The trainer decided that it was better to mail the material at the beginning of summer, so the mailing went out in mid-June. By the time the people received the mailing, their minds were no longer on getting in shape for summer. It was already summer. They had either started a fitness program or they had given up on being in shape for this summer.

Needless to say, the response was less than good. However, the offer and the material were very good. I suggested the same program be done again the following April, which it was, and it was very successful. I also had the trainer adapt the program for an October mailing to get in shape for the holidays. It too, was successful.

The moral of this story is to watch your calendar. Send your mailings so they coincide with the known preferred buying cycles of people where health and fitness is concerned.

Principle #6: Make Sense of Your Dollars

This principle of direct mail magic is very simple. Have a budget for the campaign and stick to it. Know how much your list will cost, know the cost of postage, stationery, printing, overhead, and anything else that goes into the campaign. If you cannot afford to conduct a direct mail campaign properly, do not do it. You also should not do a mailing on "spec", which is the hope that enough people will respond and join to pay for the mailing and make it profitable.

Design your budget and stay within it. You can be very successful this way, especially since you are beginning with a small market test.

Principle #7: Have Your Answer Ready

You should have your follow-up system already in place before you send out the mailing. If you have to answer telephone inquiries, mail out brochures in response to coupons, provide tours, give free supervised workouts, or make presentations to interested respondents, you must be totally prepared.

One of the worst things you can do is conduct your mailing and have no way to follow up on it. Fulfillment is critical to the success of your direct mail campaign. People who responded will become discouraged about your service and will not want to do business with you. Then, they will start to tell their friends, and there is very little a fitness director can do to overcome negative word of mouth. So, make sure you are prepared to answer all the inquiries that come from your direct mail campaign.

These seven basic principles of direct mail marketing will help you be more successful than if you just take a shotgun approach. Follow these recommendations. Begin with a small test market and as your success grows, expand your mailing areas. Each time you do another mailing, you may want to test something different in your direct mail piece.

Let's say you want to mail to two different zip codes on opposite sides of your city. You can send one offer, headline or price to one group and a different set of information to the other. Or, you can keep everything the same and vary just one aspect of the mailing, such as the price or the headline. I recommend the latter approach to testing direct mail pieces. This is because if you vary two or more items, you have no way of actually knowing what caused the response. Keep your tests of your mailings simple and controllable.

You must constantly test your direct mail pieces. Test one mailing against another to see which delivers the best response. Use the winner as your control and develop another direct mail piece. Vary one item at a time in this second piece, such as the headline, the price of your fitness program or service, or your offer. Again, determine which piece pulls better and select that as your control. After four or five tests, if you have one piece that continues to out perform the others, use it until the responses and inquiries start to dry up.

Direct mail is a very important part of direct marketing. It is probably the most well known, but there are other direct marketing methods you can use to improve your fitness business. All of them must make some type of offer to your potential customer. There are several basic principles that will make your offer very motivating. Here are some of them. Try to adapt them for your own use. Then, we will discuss other direct marketing methods.

Direct Marketing Offers

It is true that the headline of your direct marketing piece, letter, brochure or flyer, is quite often what captures someone's attention. However, if you can make them a great offer, you can even save a weak headline. These guidelines for making offers will assist you in improving the quality of your direct marketing campaigns.

There are basically three types of offers you can make, and they all should appeal to satisfying some basic need like security, receiving a reward or respect for authority. They are discounts, including free trials, special assistance, and guarantees. Some clubs go so far as to make all three offers in a single marketing communication. There is nothing wrong with that approach as long as you can fulfill your promises.

Discounts can be offered to customers who pay cash, who pay by a certain date, who buy several products or services at one time, or who purchase multiple memberships in your club. Discounts can be extended to their ultimate level by offering something for free, such as a free trial program or a free short-term membership.

Special assistance offers provide people with the knowledge that they will receive help. You may offer financing for memberships, accept credit cards, provide totally supervised workouts, accept trade-ins on other club memberships, extend current memberships for specific reasons, or even provide valet parking or taxi service.

Guarantees are very powerful offers. The most powerful of these is the unconditional, money-back guarantee if the customer is not completely satisfied. This type of guarantee is also known as risk reversal, where you are assuming all the risk. You see this a great deal with magazine and book publishers. They send you a publication that you can keep for 15 or 30 days to decide if you like it. If not, you can send it back to them. They have assumed all the risk by allowing you to "own" and try their product for a period of time.

Adapt this approach to your fitness business. Allow people to participate in your programs for free for a specified period of time. State this boldly in your direct mail offer. The word FREE is a powerful motivator. Offer **FREE MEMBERSHIPS**, **FREE PROGRAM PARTICIPATION FOR ONE WEEK**, or anything else you can think of.

Another type of guarantee is the "guaranteed, discount renewal rate". Although this may seem like a hard-core sales closing technique, if it is worded properly in your direct mail piece, it can increase your response levels.

If you are having trouble developing an offer for a direct marketing program, go back and review what you are offering. Re-evaluate your fitness programs, products or services. Brainstorm with others about the best offer to make and the best way to make it. Remember that the best offer is the one that motivates your target market to act.

Other Direct Marketing Methods

There are several other direct marketing methods you should consider. The one that is most familiar to people is the newsletter. It is a great way to keep everyone informed about your club, your corporate fitness center, your personal training business, your aerobics studio, your hospital wellness center, or your fitness consulting business. Here are some tips to help you publish a successful newsletter.

1. ***Keep it an information piece.*** Provide your readers with information about fitness and health, advances in the medical field that affect them, news about the readers themselves, and talk about your employees. DO NOT SELL in your newsletter. The fact that you are providing information informs people that you are an expert and they will know to come to you if they need what you are providing.

2. ***Make it easy to read.*** Use type sizes that are large enough for your audience to read easily, keep the sentences and the paragraphs short, use graphics and illustrations to complement the text, and use two to three columns. People are used to reading newspapers in columns and this skill will transfer over to your newsletter. Don't reinvent the wheel. Use what you know works in other areas.

3. ***Publish on time.*** Whatever schedule you develop for the newsletter, make certain you stick to it. If it is monthly, quarterly or annually, or whatever, publish on time. Your readers will be expecting it, especially if they like what you have to say.

4. ***Quality vs. Quantity.*** It is not necessary to publish a four or eight page newsletter for it to be effective. I work with someone who sends out a quarterly, one page, two column newsletter as a self mailer to all his personal training clients. It is extremely effective. Say what you have to say in as small a space as possible. People will appreciate your quality rather than your quantity.

5. ***Make a free offer.*** Since I already told you not to sell anything within the newsletter, make a free offer. This will not be perceived as selling and will be appreciated by your readers.

6. ***Use inserts.*** If your newsletter is four or more pages, use inserts. These are free standing pages that tell another story. This story can be completely different from the content of the newsletter. The insert does not have to be a story at all. It can be a blatant advertisement to sell something.

   This is not contradictory to what I said originally about not selling in the newsletter. The insert is perceived as a completely separate piece from the newsletter proper. Readers will welcome the opportunity to purchase something from the insert, especially if the offer is discounted. And, the integrity of the newsletter is still intact.

7. ***Give it away.*** This may sound like silly advice, but if you are using the newsletter to promote your club, services or products, you should give it away for free. You even pay for the postage. Now, if you are trying to start a subscription newsletter, whose information content is more general, that is another story. But, if it is just a membership/client newsletter, make sure you foot the bill and give it away.

   These seven tips will help make your newsletter much more successful. The attempt here was not to give you a course on desktop publishing. Rather, I wanted you to learn how to publish and use a successful newsletter without having to make the mistakes others have made. Now, here is an interesting twist on the newsletter idea as a direct marketing piece.

Letter of News

You probably send out correspondence to your customers or members on a regular basis. Now you can add another piece called a letter of news. This is basically the same thing as the newsletter, but it is written in a personalized letter format. You can use similar subheadings as you would in the newsletters, and you can cover different topics.

Some people get a variety of newsletters to read, and many of those never actually get read. Your personalized letter of news, however, will definitely get read because its appearance is the same as a personal letter. Keep the tone of the letter very friendly and you will find that you can make offers, sell items, and even ask people for referrals in this letter of news.

Brochures and Flyers

These are two other direct marketing pieces that you can use. They can be included in a direct mail campaign, they can be given out directly to people at various meetings, functions and places, or they can be left on cars in parking lots (with permission). Brochures and flyers provide potential customers with important information about your fitness business in a capsulized form. They may be brief, but they should be powerful and motivating.

When you create your brochures and flyers, make certain they look good and are eye-appealing. Also, make certain they sell the benefits of whatever you are trying to sell. Forget the features. People are only interested in benefits, and since you do not have much space on these pieces, you must identify the benefits you want to sell and then sell them to the hilt.

Another suggestion for developing your brochures. Many clubs and programs decide to write and design their own brochures and then take them to a quick printer to save money. Well, you do save money, but my experience is that your brochure is not nearly as well done as it can be. People find it inherently difficult to brag about themselves, and therefore they rarely develop a brochure that is as good as one developed by an outside, objective professional.

If you want a quality brochure, regardless of your budget, seek professional assistance. Graphics artists, marketing consultants, copywriters, and others who have experience in preparing brochures can help you make your brochure a winner. Remember that your brochure, and your flyer, must sell for you when you are not there.

You can also get this professional assistance for free. Offer to trade out a membership, or product, or program participation for their cooperation in helping you develop brochures. You will find that barter is an excellent marketing technique in many areas.

Direct Marketing Creativity

Don't, for one minute, think that your direct marketing efforts and direct mail pieces have to be of the standard everyday, normal routine variety. Just because your competitors send out similar pieces does not mean you have to follow suit.

The more creative you are with your direct marketing efforts, the greater your chances for success. Some creative ideas include different types of envelopes or packaging for your pieces. Or, you may want to try some of these concepts.

If you own a health club or wellness center, why not mail a plastic dumbbell to prospects. Imprint a message on the dumbbell. You will be pleasantly surprised at the response you will get.

Also, mail them a bio-dot or stress dot card - the ones that change color to tell you how much pressure you are under. Imprint the card with your name and telephone number and an invitation to call you. Again, your responses will surprise you.

Need another creative idea? Mail prospects a box with a note saying they just won a pair of athletic shoes from your facility. Include only one shoe in the box, along with your facility name and telephone number. Your prospects will call you to inform you that there was one shoe in the box. Tell them you are sorry and invite them in for the other shoe. Once they are in your facility, offer them a tour, a free one or two week membership for the inconvenience, and then sell them on a longer membership.

What other creative direct marketing ideas can you come up with? Stop limiting yourself to traditional thinking, open up your mind and you will be surprised at your results.

Telemarketing

Telemarketing is an excellent way to make your direct marketing campaign successful and profitable. Telemarketing is nothing more than calling people up on the phone, explaining to them who you are and the purpose of your call, and making them the same offer you would make in print. The key to success in telemarketing is the same as it is in other types of marketing. You must select your target market, identify and satisfy their needs, and make them an offer they find irresistible.

When using telemarketing as a marketing and sales tool, people often raise the question about a telephone script. Should one be developed and used, or should telemarketers just "wing it". Here is my suggestion, and I have found it to produce successful telemarketing campaigns in a variety of industries, including fitness.

There are two types of telemarketing scripts: formal and informal. A formal script details everything the telemarketer must say on each particular call. There can be no deviation from this script. The telemarketer also may have a flow chart to identify where to go next in the script if the person being called responds in a certain way.

Formal scripts should definitely be used for new telemarketers to your fitness business, regardless of their experience, and for inexperienced telemarketers whom you are training. Also, if a formal script has been successful in the past in attracting new members to your facility or participants to your program, then it should continue to be used by everyone.

An informal telemarketing script is basically an outline of what should be said on the phone. Informal scripts should only be used by experienced and successful telemarketers. These scripts allow the telemarketer to inject his or her own personality and experiences into the call and tend to make the call more personal.

The one thing you should never allow to happen is for someone to say whatever they want to say, rather than what they are supposed to say. All telemarketers should be giving out the same information and making the same offers. If this needs to be done through a formal script with no deviation, then do it this way. It is better for your marketing efforts to have everyone saying and doing the same thing in a "mechanical" fashion than to have employees giving out different, or possibly, wrong information.

The same concept holds true for people answering your incoming calls. They, too, are telemarketers, and they must be prepared to answer the phone properly as well as respond to any questions or situations that may arise.

Here is a hint for an effective way to answer the telephone at your facility. Always answer before the fourth ring. Then have the person say "Good morning (afternoon, evening), ABC Health Club. This is Richard. HOW may I help you?"

Answering in this way motivates the caller to provide you with more information about their call. If you answer "Can I help you?", the caller can just say no. When you speak with people, either on the phone or in person, always try to use statements, phrases or questions that will elicit more information from them. This way, you reduce the possibility of a miscommunication.

If the caller must be placed on hold, explain to the caller why they are being placed on hold and ask them if they mind. If you have to transfer the caller to someone else, tell them it will be your pleasure to do so.

These few hints on telemarketing and answering the telephone will help you be more successful in your direct marketing efforts.

One Last Thought On Direct Marketing

I mentioned earlier that typical responses to direct marketing are about 1 or 2%. Never believe everything you read or hear. You can create increased responses simply by following up your direct marketing piece with a personal telephone call. In fact, use a technique called response compression and you will possibly increase your response rate over 5 or 10%.

Response compression works like this. It involves multiple contacts with a prospect within a short period of time, say two weeks. For example, you mail a piece to a prospect on a Monday, call them on Friday to make certain they received the piece, mail them another piece on Monday, call again on Wednesday, and call again on Friday. The purpose of all these contacts is for you to try to schedule an appointment with the prospect or to get them to visit your facility, and to begin to develop a relationship with this person. Remember that the more familiar you are to them, the greater the chances of their doing business with you.

MAKE ALL YOUR MARKETING AND ADVERTISING DIRECT RESPONSE!!!

Implementing a Public Relations Campaign

Chapter 5

Using Public Relations to Increase Marketing Success

There are a great many "experts" who think they know exactly what public relations is, and they will be glad to tell you. Usually, it costs you. Some of these experts will tell you that public relations doesn't cost anything, and that is wrong. Some of these experts will tell you that public relations is simply sending out press releases, and that is wrong.

Public relations is much more than either of these things. PR, as it is called, is the sum total of all your efforts that results in publicity for you and your facility or programs. Sometimes, it is free, but more often there are some costs associated with it. These costs include time, personnel, effort, paper, materials, travel, and everything else that you put into getting that dose of publicity.

An Example of Good Public Relations

Let me give you an example of good public relations, and then we will go into how to develop your PR campaign. A fitness center was about to open in a highly competitive, urban area. They did not have an extensive marketing or advertising budget, like their mega-chain competitors, nor did they have much knowledge about how to generate publicity. They were great at providing health and fitness programs and services, but not at marketing. Here is what we did for them.

First, we convinced them to have a "soft" opening. A soft opening is when you open the facility with a minimum of advertising, publicity and hype. Your goal is to "get the kinks out", get your systems in place, and make certain your staff is trained. We had them stay "soft" for 30 days, which gave us enough time to plan their **Grand Opening**.

For the grand opening, we had a budget of a few hundred dollars. This is basically nothing, so we decided to donate it to a local charity. The charity was contacted and asked to send a representative to the opening. Then, news directors and assignment editors at the radio and television stations were called and sent a letter about the upcoming public donation. These people were invited to attend and cover the story as well as the grand opening.

Next, we sent press releases to all the media about the grand opening three weeks before the date, two weeks and one week prior to the event. We also called them. We made certain the media knew the opening was going to happen. Then, we found a local talk radio

35

station that had a health-related show on it. We convinced the hosts to hold their show "live" from the facility on that day. They mentioned their remote broadcast for several weeks prior to the event, which helped increase the turnout.

Since we had no money to advertise, we had to do something to inform the rest of the public. We worked with several radio stations and "traded out" advertising time for membership. While there may be a way to equate costs associated with a trade out of this type, there really is no way to place a price on the value the fitness center received from the "free" advertising on the radio. Because more than one station aired the commercials, the public perceived that this was a well financed operation.

The grand opening was a tremendous success. The center converted 30% of the people who came that day, and has re-signed 75% of those people who received free, initial memberships. The total financial cost to the facility was only the $300 they donated to the charity, and it was tax deductible.

A Review of The Public Relations For The Event

Let's quickly review the public relations activites that were conducted for this event. First, there was a charity tie-in. The media loves to cover charity events and donations to charities. The incremental exposure from this alone was worth over $10,000.00. Next, press releases were sent and telephone calls made to the media about the charity donation at the grand opening. This led to additional coverage. Third, a local radio talk show conducted their show live from the facility, which led to even more free promotion. Fourth, free advertising was received through membership trade outs. Finally, once the grand opening was over, we sent out a press release telling everyone about the tremenously successful event.

Can You Apply These Techniques To Your Facility?

The answer to this question is a rousing YES!! Just adapt them, or follow them to the letter for any event you want to hold at your facility. They have worked in the past in the fitness industry as well as for other companies in other industries. There is no reason why the approach should not work for you now.

Also, modify the techniques to suit your needs. You know what is best for your facility, and you know the type of publicity you want to gain. Now, just go out and get the coverage you need to publicize yourself.

Here are some helpful hints.

The Purpose of Public Relations

The purpose of public relations is simply to get media coverage, preferably at little or no cost to you, for your fitness facility and programs. A secondary purpose is to establish community goodwill and positive community relations. Here are some ways to generate that publicity.

Press Releases

Press releases are the most common method for informing the media about what you are doing. Many books will tell you to follow a basic format for writing the press release, which includes putting the words "NEWS RELEASE" in the upper right hand corner, the date, contact person and telephone number on the left margin, and the words, "FOR IMMEDIATE RELEASE" flush right. The sample format on the next page shows this to you graphically.

Then, you highlight and/or capitalize the title of the release, skip two lines and put the city and state associated with the release, and begin your message. Remember to double space between lines. Also, your release should read from the specific to the general, and answer the questions: who, what, when, where, how and why. Editors may use all of your release, they may rewrite it, or they may use portions of it. When they start to edit it, they usually do so from the bottom up. Therefore, put your most important information at the beginning of the release.

This basic format is successful for many people, and I recommend you use it. The sample on the next page gives you an idea of a one page release. Try to keep your press releases to one or two pages. If you go to two pages, place -MORE- at the bottom of the first page. On the last page, end the release with the symbol -30- or ###. This tells an editor that the material is finished.

Now, understand that many fitness directors, and people in other industries, are sending press releases to the same people you are, and they are using the same or a similar format. Maybe, just to make sure your release gets read, you should consider being a little creative with your format. Write the release in the form of a newspaper article, as mentioned previously, so they can publish it as is if they want to. Or, write it with some graphics included in it. Or, reverse out the headline and use white print on a black background. Whatever you do, be creative.

NEWS RELEASE

DATE:
CONTACT: Richard F. Gerson
TELEPHONE: (813) 726-7619

FOR IMMEDIATE RELEASE

NEW MARKETING BOOK PUBLISHED
EXCLUSIVELY FOR FITNESS DIRECTORS

Safety Harbor, Florida - Professional Reports Corporation is pleased to announce the publication to their newest book, **The Fitness Director's Guide to Marketing Strategies and Tactics**, by Richard F. Gerson, Ph.D. This is the eighth book written by Dr. Gerson and the second on marketing for the health/fitness industry.

The book covers the entire range of marketing efforts, including marketing planning, advertising, public relations, promotions, customer service and selling. Dr. Gerson provides the reader with over 130 low cost or no cost marketing techniques that can be used to effectively promote a fitness business, along with over 50 customer service tips.

Dr. Gerson is considered one of the premier marketing consultants in the country, and is the leading expert in fitness marketing. He has provided numerous seminars at regional and national conventions for the industry, and there have always been overflowing crowds. This book is an excellent addition to any fitness director's library, especially if they are interested in successfully marketing their club, wellness center, personal training, health promotion, or consulting business.

For more information on the book or to order it, contact Professional Reports Corporation at 1-800-336-0083. Dr. Gerson can be reached at 813-726-7619 or by writing to P.O. Box 1534, Safety Harbor, Florida 34695. He is available as a consultant, trainer and speaker.

# # #

Charities and Charity Tie-Ins

Every fitness business should be associated with a local charity, or a local chapter of a national organization. The publicity you receive from this alliance is tremendous. You can publicize it, and the charity will definitely publicize it. Hold fundraisers for the charity, do special events, volunteer for their committees and boards, and even host open houses for their volunteers. Do anything and everything you can for a charity and the media will love you.

Other Publicity Opportunities

One of the purposes of public relations is to create a public perception of you as an expert, or your facility or programs as the one to attend. You need to constantly be in the public's eye and reinforce in their minds all the wonderful things you can do for them at your facility or through your programs. Here are some additional ideas you can use to create the image of you as an expert while at the same time generating publicity for your facility and programs. Those ideas that were mentioned earlier in the book are repeated here to emphasize their importance.

Publish

Write articles. It is as simple as that. Call up your local weekly newspaper, or some other publication, and offer to write articles for them on health and fitness. You do not have to be paid for writing. All you want is a byline and a brief biography at the end of the article. The more articles you write, the more the public will see your name and face (send a picture to the publication) and start to consider you as an expert.

You can also write for your trade publications. There are over two dozen trade publications, and just as many professional publications, in the health and fitness field. Find out what they are, write a letter or call the editor, tell the editor who you are and your qualifications, and then describe the article you want to write. OR, write the article and send it in unsolicited and hope they print it.

How powerful is this publicity technique of publishing articles? I can tell you it works for me as I have published over 200 articles in various publications. However, let me tell you how it helped one of the country's best-known fitness consultants and motivational speakers get started.

When this gentleman asked me how he could get started publicizing himself, I suggested he publish an article. Since he had never done that before, we agreed to co-author an article on Men in Aerobics. It was the first article ever published on the subject, and my co-author was asked to speak at several conventions on this topic. As he polished his writing skills, I suggested he try to write for his local newspapers. He immediately established himself as the author of a regular fitness column in several local newspapers in the Ft. Myers/Sanibel area of Florida. He then began to publish again in magazines, and to send out press releases about his publications.

This gentleman has since gone on to much bigger and more successful things, such as being on the cover of Men's Fitness magazine, appearing on the cover and featured in American Fitness magazine, and being featured in GQ magazine. He is internationally known as a fitness expert and motivational speaker. You may have heard him. His name is David Essel. And, his monumental success all began with publishing several articles.

Remember that people believe what they see in print. The more articles you publish on health and fitness, the more of an expert the public will perceive you to be. Also, you should write your own book or booklet. Self publish it, and send out press releases that you have done so. Self publishing has achieved a level of credibility now that it never had before. As long as the information you are publishing is timely and helpful, you can tell the world you have written and published a book.

Speak

Give speeches. Do the "rubber chicken" circuit - the lunch club meetings. Get out and give as many speeches as you can, especially when you are just starting out. Also, try to speak at trade meeting and conventions.

Use your speaking abilities in another way. Speak out on certain issues related to health and fitness. Become a media resource. Contact media people and let them know you are available as an expert in the field should they have any questions.

Get interviewed. Call up local talk show hosts and offer to be a guest on their show. Talk about a timely fitness topic and always mention your affiliation with your facility or programs. These shows can be on network affiliates, cable TV, or radio.

Awards

If you get an award or a certification, publicize it. Better yet, give out an award and publicize that. The media loves to cover award ceremonies. Also, in your club, give out awards for best employee and best member and publicize these events. The more mentions you get in a newspaper, or anywhere else, as being associated with someone else receiving an award, the greater your prospects are for gaining "goodwill" business.

New Hires and Promotions

Whenever you hire someone, or promote someone, send a press release and their picture to the newspapers telling who the person is, what they have done and what they will be doing for you. Make sure you mention your company name in the press release.

This is an innocuous way of getting coverage, and the newspapers are only too happy to print good news about other people. Also, send them information on your own personal good news events.

Your Press/Publicity Kit

It seems that every fitness center or health promotion program has their own brochure. In fact, the world is inundated with brochures. Since most brochures are "me" pieces, rather than sales pieces, they tend to get thrown away. Instead of a brochure, think about developing a press or publicity kit for yourself, your facility or your programs.

I have found that the press kit is much more effective, and makes a greater impact on prospects, customers and members, than any type of brochure, no matter how expensive the brochure was to print.

Your press kit can be a folder-type binder with slip pockets and a slot for your business card, or even a three ring binder. If you use a three ring binder, as I do, make certain all the pages are in vinyl sheets. This protects the pages and makes your content last longer. Also, the reason I use a three ring binder instead of a folder is that the binder makes more of an impact on the prospect or customer. Furthermore, since I do not give them the pages from the binder, it requires that I mail them or drop off the material if they request it. This gives me another contact with them and another chance to get my name in front of them.

Here are some suggestions for what should go into your press kit.
1. Company Description. This is a one or two page description of your company, including what programs and services it offers, its customer service philosophy, and its approaches to helping customers. Keep this description positive and upbeat.
2. Personal Biography. As the owner or marketing contact for your company, people want to know with whom they are dealing. Provide information on who you are, your background and achievements, and how you plan to help your customers.
3. Client List. Provide a list of your clients or people you have done business with. For example, in a club setting or a hospital setting, you may want to list the corporations who are members or who have participated in your programs.
4. Client Benefits. Always sell the benefits, not the features. List all the benefits your customer will receive from working with you.
5. Testimonial Letters. Provide several different testimonial letters that sing your praises. The more letters you can provide, the more people perceive you are an expert.
6. Program Descriptions. Describe the programs and services you offer. If possible, write an outline of any training programs and also a list of benefits that people will receive from attending these programs.
7. Publications. Provide samples or reprints of any articles you authored. People enjoy doing business with published authors. This also enhances your credibility.

These are the contents of a press kit. You should also include your business card, and black and white photos of you. Press kits can accompany press releases, requests for more information about you or your company, or they can be sent along with business proposals. In any case, the press kit must sell you to the reader in order for you to gain publicity and eventually, more business.

Sponsorships

Another great public relations opportunity, and an excellent marketing tool, is a sponsorship of a local athletic team, youth group, senior group, or special event. Although this may cost you some money, the return on your investment is tremendous. You build community good will along with getting your name out in front of the public.

Some things you can sponsor include little league teams, soccer teams, high school athletic events, community dances, fund raisers, special trips or outings, a cub/girl scout troop, charity events, races, aerobic dance marathons, and anything else you can think of.

Cultivating Your Public Relations

People often wonder why their press releases do not get printed, their event announcements do not receive any coverage, and the media seems uninterested in what they are doing. It is not because your health or fitness event is without merit. You must remember that media people always have a full plate, and your press release must be extremely newsworthy to get through to them and warrant coverage. Here is how to increase your chances of getting media coverage.

Take an editor to lunch! It's true. Call up your local newspaper editor, news director, assignment editor, or whomever has the authority to decide whether or not you will receive media coverage. Tell them you want to meet them personally to introduce yourself and you would like to do this over lunch, or breakfast, or dinner. If they politely refuse, ask them if you can come to their office to meet them and to drop off some material that might interest them.

Keep in regular contact with them. When you have something newsworthy, call them up and offer them an exclusive on your event. If you offer an exclusive, never provide the information to another medium until your first one has either covered it or rejected it.

Send them letters thanking them for coverage. Send them items of interest from the health and fitness field. Keep in touch with them even when you do not have anything newsworthy for them. In fact, this may get you more coverage because they will perceive that every time they hear from you, it's not just for publicity. If you cannot become their friend, at least be friendly.

Also, don't send press releases to them or call them with every little thing that comes up. You will be labeled as a publicity hound. Only contact the media when there is something that they perceive will interest their audience. And that is how you must present it: as something of interest to their audience. The less self serving you appear to be, the greater your chance for publicity.

Last, But Not Least

One more thing about public relations and publicity. Put yourself on a regular schedule for the year to inform the public about your newsworthy accomplishments or events. This can be monthly, bi-monthly quarterly, bi-annually or annually. Just make sure you stick to this schedule and the material you send in, or the events you sponsor or host, are newsworthy enough to warrant free media coverage.

Never become like the boy who cried wolf, and send press releases or make telephone calls every time someone changes their socks. Make your requests for media coverage important enough to warrant space, and beneficial enough to the audience so that the media person feels comfortable giving you that free space.

Also, you must remember that sending out press releases involves postage costs, so be judicious with what you mail. Target your media markets as carefully as you target your customer markets. Nurture them in the same way as you do your customers to grow your publicity efforts to where the media is glad to hear from you. Then, publicize, publicize, publicize, and keep all the above principles in mind.

Advertising For Success

Chapter 6

How To Get Twice The Advertising At Half The Cost
IF YOU ARE WORKING WITH AN ADVERTISING AGENCY, FIRE THEM!!

I cannot make this statement any more emphatically. There are many reasons you should not work with an ad agency. Here are my top five:

1. Most ad agencies create an ad campaign, advertising plan or media plan with little or no knowledge or regard for *your* marketing plan.
2. Most ad campaigns are designed to showcase the creative talents of the agencies and possibly win awards rather than increase your sales and revenue.
3. Most ad agencies know nothing about marketing, and less about fitness marketing.
4. Advertising works best with mass market, consumer oriented products, and you are not in that business.
5. If your account is small, and it typically will be, you will receive the least amount of attention from the agency from their least skilled and qualified employees and account executives.

All these reasons combine to have me tell you again to fire your advertising agency. You can do just as well, and I think even better, by creating your own campaign and working with a marketing consultant and freelance artists and writers to create the visual and written aspects of your ads.

One of the reasons for my success as a marketing consultant has been my ability to go into fitness centers and other companies, review their advertising campaigns, make specific recommendations that are more marketing-oriented, rewrite their copy, and then turn the ad into a piece that will sell.

That is your ultimate goal. If you do any advertising at all, it must be salesmanship in print, or on the radio or television. You cannot, and should not even try to afford an image building ad campaign or an institutional advertising campaign. Leave that for the mega-corporations with money to burn. You need to make every dollar you spend on communicating with the public generate at least 10 times its value.

Now, don't get me totally wrong. I am not against advertising. I am against advertising for the sake of advertising and winning awards rather than creating sales.

Did you know that when a survey was done on the "still running bunny" for Everready batteries, 90% of the people remembered seeing that ad. The unfortunate thing was that they thought it was an ad for Duracell, a major competitor. Consequently, sales of Duracell batteries increased while sales for Everready remained the same or slightly decreased.

Or, one company that shall remain nameless, totally rejected an ad agency's campaign for them. The agency submitted the campaign for an award anyway, and they won. This is a sad state of affairs when advertising that a client would not accept is still capable of winning an award.

There are situations when advertising does work and does generate sales and revenue. These situations usually occur when the ad campaign is based on the company's marketing strategy and supports the marketing and sales efforts geared to a target market. For example, assume you developed a new program for seniors and wanted to communicate with them the benefits of this exercise program.

An ad agency may have you take out a big ad in the local major newspaper, place ads on radio stations these people listen to, and possibly conduct a direct mail program to them. An ad agency that works from a marketing perspective, or a marketing consultant, will have you forget the major newspaper and the radio station for now. You should advertise in the senior newspapers and the shopper guides that your target market reads. You should deliver flyers to their communities and also give speeches at their residences. These are much more effective and definitely less expensive ways to inform your senior target market of your new exercise program for them.

That is what the rest of this chapter is about: How you can make your advertising twice as effective for much less money than you may be used to paying.

10 Common Myths About Advertising

Experience has taught us that people believe the following 10 common myths about advertising. Fortunately, these beliefs have all been exposed as myths and now you can learn from other people's mistakes.

1. *Advertising has to be expensive to be effective.* Nothing can be further from the truth. There are many creative and inventive ways to get free advertising that works. There are also many promotional techniques that can be used as advertising to increase your sales.

2. *Advertising is too expensive for the fitness club owner or fitness service provider.* Just as in number 1, you can create advertising campaigns that are very effective for very little money. Also, you may want to think about trading out some of your memberships to consultants, writers or artists to help you develop your advertising campaign.

3. *Advertising is what you must do to get business.* Advertising is only one of many ways to get business. In fact, there are many more ways to get your business than advertising. The key is to keep the business once you have it.

4. *One shot, one big hit ad, is all that's needed.* Advertising is not a one shot deal. That is why they call it an advertising campaign. It is something that must be developed and used over a period of time. Furthermore, you must realize that it takes between 7 and 21 advertising impressions for a person to begin to remember who you are and what you do. This concept is based on the rule of 7's, which states that a message must be noticed

by a potential customer at least 7 times before any action is taken on it. Plus, it takes at least 3 tries to get a customer to notice you in the first place. Therefore, you must make between 7 and 21 advertising impressions to start being successful. However, it only takes one impression when that comes from a credible referral source.

5. ***There is one best advertising approach or method.*** Advertising is nothing more than an experiment, a crap shoot. The ad can look or sound great, everyone involved with its creation may think its great, the medium you place it in thinks its great, and the customers do not pay any attention to it. Plus, fitness directors and club owners sometimes get caught in a trap because of their limited ad budgets and decide to put all their money into one approach. That's like investing your life savings in a new company's stock and hoping against hope you won't go broke.

Successful advertising is based on testing, testing and retesting. And, you must test different advertising mediums. Therefore, never put all your eggs (money) in one basket (approach). Even if it works for you for a while, you can get lulled into a false sense of security. Try a variety of approaches, see which one works the best for a given target market, then invest more time and money in that approach.

6. ***Advertising does your work for you.*** No one can afford to sit back and wait for advertising to work. What if it doesn't? Then what do you do?

Advertising is merely one of several ways to get business, and it is a passive way at that. You must develop active marketing and advertising techniques that will support your passive advertising. You must work so that the advertising will work also.

7. ***Short ad copy is better (more effective) than long copy.*** This is one of the biggest myths about advertising and direct mail. People will read copy of any length, as long as they are interested in it. Reading interest tends to drop off between 50 and 500 words, so if you can keep them interested through two pages of copy, you've got them hooked.

The reason people do not read long ads is because they are not interested in the content. This is usually the result of a weak headline or poor supporting copy, or the copy telling the story of the advertiser without emphasizing any benefits for the reader, listener or viewer. You must write all your copy, regardless of whether it is short or long, from the perspective of the customer. Consider the features of what you are selling, the advantages to the customer, and the benefits they will receive.

8. ***Advertising generally attracts new customers.*** The fact is that advertising more often reminds current or former customers why they should continue to do business with you. Your other marketing and promotional techniques do more to generate new business than advertising.

9. ***Advertising is most effective when it is image advertising.*** Every business, fitness or otherwise, wants to project a positive and popular public image. The truth is that most businesses cannot afford an image advertising campaign. Unfortunately, most ads are developed to promote an image rather than to sell a service. Just look at your typical club ads. They usually show a well built male or female (possibly the unattainable body for the general public) with a specific offer regarding membership. The image that is portrayed is one of beautiful people, and if that is what your facility wants to be perceived as, great. However, if your facility wants to be perceived as successful, and actually be

successful, then you need to stop any and all image advertising and develop direct response, sales-oriented advertising.

10. ***Advertising determines the success of a business.*** Again, this is completely false. There are many businesses that do no formal advertising and are extremely successful. My own consulting business is a case in point. We never pay for advertising of any kind, anywhere. If you have ever seen an ad of ours in a magazine, it is the result of a trade out for an article I have written or some work I conducted for the publication. The success of my business is totally dependent on marketing and promotions. The same will hold true for your fitness business.

You can use advertising to influence the success of your business, but only if the advertising is based on your marketing plan. Develop a marketing plan for your facility, use the strategies and tactics you will find throughout and in the back of this book, and then develop your advertising to support the marketing plan, strategies and tactics.

I must clarify one other myth related to advertising and business success. Many people erroneously believe that only good advertising agencies can create successful ads. Forget it. I have deliberately never worked with an ad agency to create ads for my clients, and you don't have to either. Audition artists and copywriters, or other freelancers that you may need, and have them help you develop your ads. You will find that the campaigns you create equal or exceed whatever the "good" or big agency could have created, and at a fraction of the cost.

Now that we have exposed some of the most common myths about advertising, let's discuss how to develop successful ads and then where to place them.

How To Develop a Successful/Effective Ad

Start with the headline. This is the most important part of any ad. If your headlines do not scream a benefit to the reader, why should that person take the time to read the rest of your ad. Too many fitness centers, and other businesses (even those working with ad agencies), advertise with a warm fuzzy headline that looks, sounds or feels nice. Unfortunately, it does not get the reader to continue with the rest of the ad.

For example, many clubs and wellness centers advertise new year membership specials for the monthly price of the new year number (Join now for only $19.92 a month) or weight loss programs at their facilities as people try to keep their resolutions to lose weight. Look at that "Join now" headline. It is not exciting, it does not motivate anyone, except maybe someone who is shopping for a cheap price, and it does not make me want to read further because it is the same as every other ad.

Ask yourself these questions. Who is it that you want to join now? Identify your target market and make the headline suit them. Direct it right toward them. Also, what is it that your target market really wants? You can put this benefit in the headline or in a sub-headline. Finally, how can you support the benefit claims you made in the headline? This is where you must write great body copy to motivate the reader to call you or come into your facility.

Try this approach, and feel free to adapt the following example to your situation. Notice how the headline screams a benefit and the rest of the sample ad supports that benefit.

Your club has decided to attract the baby boomers who are just turning forty. Research shows us that this group of consumers will not age gracefully, they will fight it all the way. The research also shows that baby boomers are returning to former values, such as nostalgia, family, friends, and the way it was. You can combine this information, their fighting the aging process, returning to things past, and wanting to be with their families, into the following ad.

"You Can Look and Feel 25 Again"
Now there is no need to feel your age. Just because you are 40 or older does not mean you have reached middle age. In fact, you are younger now than any other generation who has reached 40 before you. Our exercise and fitness programs can help you get into better shape than you were 15 or 20 years ago. And we will do it for you at prices that are 15 or 20 years old, only $10 a month. So, if you really are 40 years old, or just feel like you're getting older, CALL xxx-xxxx today and we will start you on your way to feeling great and looking younger NOW. And, your family can join with you for only an additional $xx.xx ... a month. Call today. xxx-xxxx.

This ad covers everything we just mentioned about the headline and supporting copy. The headline screams a benefit that is specific to your target market and the copy supports that benefit. You identify a problem in the ad and then give the reader a solution. Finally, you tell them to call now to receive this benefit. Let's discuss each of these actions separately.

Body Copy

After you have written the headline, you must write the copy of the ad. Here's a hint. The headline can be written last, after the copy has been written. I have seen too many instances where people try to develop their own ads and begin with a headline that does not say anything. Actually, their headline is buried in their copy, usually within the first three or four lines. So, sometimes you may want to write your copy and then search it for your headline.

Here is a real life example. A hospital wellness center wanted to develop a back care program for its members and the general public as part of its health promotion offerings. The staff created an ad that was headlined "Back Care Program offered at ABC Wellness Center". Does that excite you or does it look like every other ad you've seen for back programs?

When they asked me to revise the ad and make it a selling ad, I found their headline in the second sentence. After some editing, their headline became "Your Back Does Not Have to Hurt Anymore!" This screams at back pain suffers that there is a way to get relief. The copy then went on to tell the reader how to ease the pain and suffering, how to join the program, and how to get in touch with the center.

I suggested to the fitness director that the next time they write their own ads, write the entire ad first before trying to put a headline on it. Once the ad was written, check out the copy. Make sure the copy is geared to the target market the facility was trying to attract, then search the copy for a powerful benefit statement that could be used as a headline.

Here are a few other points about writing the body copy. You do not always have to follow proper grammatical rules. Copy does not have to be written in perfect sentences. In fact, you may want to consider writing in short, choppy, incomplete sentences. That is how people read the fastest and understand the best. Also, feel free to leave out punctuation marks such as periods and commas. Don't worry how the copy would look to your high school English teacher. The only concern you should have is if the copy is powerful and motivating enough to get someone to respond. Again, the ad must be salesmanship in print.

Calls to Action

Every ad must have a call to action. This is where you tell the reader to contact you, either by telephone, mail or in person. Make your call to action as visible and direct as possible. You want the reader, or listener or viewer, to respond immediately to you.

In print advertising, tell them to call or write or visit in big, bold letters. On radio, use music as a background and change the tone of the announcer's voice. On television, use graphics and other visuals to emphasize your call to action.

Coding and Tracking

You must be able to code and track all your advertising. If you do not know where your business is coming from, how will you know how effective your efforts are.

Coding is a simple process of placing an extension number on the telephone number in the ad, having the respondent call and ask for a specific person, putting a coupon in the ad with a specific end date, or using a key that only you understand in an unobtrusive part of the printed ad (such as, A101).

The code you use helps you track the effectiveness of your advertising. This way, you can determine your return on investment. If you are advertising and it is costing you $2000 a month, but you are only selling $1000 a month worth of memberships, you are losing half your investment. Now, don't think that the $1000 can be considered image advertising. Remember that I said earlier most businesses and clubs cannot afford image advertising. Plain and simple, you are losing money.

If you advertise in a variety of places, each ad must have its own code, especially if the ads are identical. You must be able to determine exactly how much revenue each ad placement is generating. Then, you can decide if you want to continue with that advertising.

Be careful of the coding and tracking trap other clubs and businesses fall into. Coding and tracking takes a little bit more effort, not much, but a little bit. Yet, people don't want to expend that effort, so they just bypass these activities. Then, when it comes time to evaluate the effectiveness of their marketing and advertising programs, they can't. That's the trap I hope you will avoid. Code and track everything. This way, you will know if you are getting twice the advertising effectiveness for half the cost.

Ad Placement

Many facilities are not certain whether they should use print advertising, radio or television. Each has its benefits and drawbacks. You must consider your budget, your target audience, and your marketing/advertising goals. Also, remember that you are not obligated to advertise in only one medium at a time. You can use multiple mediums to support each other and enhance your advertising efforts.

Print Advertising

There are several advantages to print advertising. The ad lasts longer than radio and television; people go back and read it; you can put a coupon in it that they have to cut out and bring to you; and it is fairly affordable. However, if your facility is in a city where there is only one major newspaper, that paper can charge you and everyone else higher than normal rates. They have no competition. Therefore, check out the smaller, neighborhood papers and see if these will reach your target markets.

The main disadvantage of print advertising is that you do not know how many people actually read your ad. Don't believe the paper's circulation numbers. While they may sell that many papers, you can be sure all the buyers are not reading your ad. In fact, there is research that says people only see ads they are consciously or subconsciously looking for. If that is the case, then most readers of a paper or magazine will never even see your ad.

Print advertising is sold on a space basis. Your ad size is based on column inches. This means that your ad will be a certain number of columns wide by "X" number of inches long. Multiply the two numbers to get your column inches. The price is then calculated accordingly.

You can get a better price on your ads by asking for a contract rate. A contract rate simply means you agree to place a certain number of column inches with the paper during the year. The more inches of advertising you place, the better your rate will be.

Be careful when negotiating your contract rate. Ask the paper what happens if you do not use up all the space you contract for. Are you liable and will you have to then pay the higher prevailing rate for the lesser number of inches? Also, does the paper require you to use a small classified ad as a rate holder? This type of ad is put in by you, it costs you money, and it guarantees the paper will hold your contract rate for you. Find this out up front. You do not want to be surprised when you receive an invoice and the price is higher than you thought it would be.

Here are some other suggestions. You do not have to provide the paper with camera ready ads. They will be more than happy to typeset and layout your ads for you for free. Additionally, most papers have artists and writers who will help you design your ads, also for free. I strongly recommend using the free typesetting and design services. I caution you about the free artists and writers. Many times, in this situation, you get what you pay for.

A final thought on print advertising. Ask for a proof of your ad before it appears and then ask for tear sheets. These requests will guarantee that your ad looks the way you want it to look and that your ad was placed on the day and in the section you requested. Keep these ads to help you improve your future ads.

Hint: Another way to improve your ads is to create a "swipe file" of competitors' ads. Clip out their print ads, find out how well they work, adapt the best elements of their ads for your next ad, and then create the "perfect ad" for your fitness business.

Radio Advertising

In some markets, radio advertising is less expensive than print advertising. When you create an ad for radio, the same principles hold about headlines, benefits, copy, selling and calls to action. Only now, you have another medium, sound, with which to convey your message. Use this to your advantage. That is why automobile ads tend to speak fast and loudly, to get your attention. Do whatever you must to get the listener's attention. You only have 15, 30 or 60 seconds.

Radio advertising is priced on the number of listeners, time of day, and the ratings of the station or the show. Ad reps will also talk to you about reach, frequency and gross rating points. These terms are simply how many people listen to a show (reach), how often (frequency), and the multiple of the two (gross rating points-GRP). Don't worry about these.

Your only concern with radio is: Does the station/show I want to advertise on have a large enough listening audience in the age/income/demographic bracket that I want to hit? If it does, ask to see their numbers from the rating services, not their own research.

Once you have decided to advertise on radio, select your show or times. Specific times may cost you more than run of schedule, which is where they put your ad on whenever they have unsold time. If you are a 24 hour club, this may not be bad because they often have unsold time in the middle of the night. These are the night owls you are trying to attract.

Whatever times you choose, have the station prepare a media buy for you, which shows you the dates, times, length of commercial/ad, and number of ads you will have during a specific time period. The buy will also show you your costs. Now, you should ask the station to match your paid for ads with free ads plus promotional one liners. These liners are statements made by the host or disc jockey that promotes your facility, and they are free.

When you ask for free matching ads, you cannot always determine when they will run. Just the fact that they will run has helped you double your advertising. You can increase its effectiveness even more by telling the station to let you know whenever they have unsold space. You may want to have them air your ad. In print advertising, this is called remnant space. The concept is not often used by clubs on the radio or TV, but you can be the first.

Radio stations will also produce your ads for free. They will even help you with the scripts and getting the talent for the voices. This saves you a lot of money. All you have to do is ask them for this service. Remember, though, to get a tape of the commercial before it airs. This is like an ad proof from the paper. You must make certain the commercial says what you want it to say in the way you want it to say it. This is especially important if the talent was supplied by the station.

Television

Television advertising costs money. There are no two ways about it. Is it worth it? That depends on what you are trying to accomplish with your advertising.

Television can reach the most amount of people in the shortest amount of time. You are paying for that premium and capability. Network advertising is more expensive than local station advertising. Cable TV is less expensive than all of them. On top of all your ad costs, you also have production costs.

Sometimes stations will work with you to produce your television commercial. If you buy enough time, they may provide a film crew for you and charge you a reduced rate. Or, they may not. In any case, TV commercials can be expensive to produce. Remember the NIKE commercial with Bugs Bunny and Michael Jordan that aired at the 1992 NBA all star game? Reports place the cost of making that commercial, nor airing it, at around $3 million. That's an unbelievable amount of money for a short time on a television screen.

If you choose to use television as an advertising medium, make your commercials as inviting, exciting and motivating as possible. Show your club and your members having a great time. Use colors, fast changing scenes, music and lots of visuals. Show activity. Activity breeds activity. And, give your telephone number and/or location two or three times during the commercial.

Ask the TV station, network or cable, to match your paid-for ads with free commercial time. If they have unsold time, they may be willing to put you on the air. Also, consider run of schedule to save some money. Another approach is to have the station edit your 30 or 60 second commercial to a 10 or 15 second one, and then use it as a filler when they have unsold time.

You will never know if you can get these extra placements unless you ask.

Yellow Pages Advertising

Your club, wellness center, training facility, or you, should be in the Yellow Pages. You receive a free one line listing just for having your business phone. Of course, the Yellow Pages representatives will try to sell you on display ads. Be careful. These cost, and if your Yellow Pages display ad is not bringing in 10 times its monthly costs in revenues, then the ad is not effective.

Before you consider a display ad, consider working with your in-column ad. Make it bolder, use larger lettering, use red ink, use a logo, or develop an in-column display ad. This will stand out once the reader gets to your page. It is also less expensive than regular display ads.

Remember that the Yellow Pages places their full page ads in a category first, then their half page, and so on down the line. That is why they want to sell you a large display ad: so you can be closer to the front of your category. Don't believe it. Full page display ads are not necessary for everyone. It depends on your type of facility and what you are selling in the ad.

If you are going to use a display ad, follow the principles for print advertising where your headline screams a benefit. Add one more thing, and that is a banner headline in reversed out print (white print on a black background) that gives away something for free. It can be a workout, a fitness evaluation, a free blood pressure test, anything with the word free in it. This will capture the reader's attention and get them to continue to read your ad.

The rest of your ad talks about either problems and solutions or benefits to the reader. Try not to list features or program names. List what their participation in these programs will do for them. Tell them how good they will look and feel, how much weight they will lose, how strong they will be, etc. Make your telephone number and location prominent and your facility name readable. However, don't make your name the headline or the largest part of the ad. In fact, this holds true for all ads. If they read about your benefits and problem solutions, and they are interested in what you are selling, they will be able to find your name in the ad.

You can have your Yellow Pages ad prepared for free by the company that is selling you the advertising. They will lay it out, design it, typeset it, and show you as many proofs as you desire before it is printed. And all this work costs you nothing. Just ask for it, and they will gladly provide the service.

Also, once your ad appears in a newspaper or your name gets listed on a licensed list or in the business section of the paper, you may be contacted by a Yellow Pages buying service. They will tell you that if you let them place your ads for you, it will cost you less. Be careful. Check this out by calling the Yellow Pages directly and getting price quotes on the same size ads. Often times, the buying service does not really save you any money. They may offer you a discount if you pay them in full (10% off when the entire year is paid in full), and this may be your only savings. You must determine if this is worth having your cash in their account, or would you rather pay the full amount of the ad directly to the Yellow Pages, but on a monthly basis? This way, your money is still working for you.

Follow the above recommendations for creating and placing your Yellow Pages and regular advertising and you will find that your ad effectiveness will double. You will essentially be getting twice the advertising for half the price. Here are a few more suggestions to help you make your advertising twice as effective.

Per Inquiry or Per Order Advertising

This is a very simple approach to advertising that allows you to advertise without paying any money up front. You work with the advertising medium to allow you to pay them on a per inquiry basis. You pay them a specified amount of money for every inquiry (call, visit or letter) you get from your ad. Or, you pay them on a per order (or per sale) basis. In either case, you have to do a masterful job of selling the advertising medium on the fact that they can make more money this way than if you paid them up front. Sometimes it works, sometimes it doesn't.

Other Unique Advertising Approaches

Everyone wants to be a star. I have never met a true fitness professional who did not want to be on a radio or television show, write his or her own column for a newspaper or magazine, or star in their own show or video. Now you can have all these things as part of your advertising program, and none of them are too expensive.

A Star is Born

You are no doubt aware of the proliferation of exercise, health and fitness videos on the market today. You can have your own video for a very reasonable cost. This video can be an exercise program starring you or it can be a corporate video selling your club, facility or wellness center. In any case, videos can be made very professionally and fairly inexpensively.

The same can be said for having your own television show. If the local network affiliates do not have a time slot for you, consider cable television. Most cable stations are looking for a fitness show or a health promotion show. Check out the costs with the station manager and learn if they will produce the show and secure advertising for you. Find out if you can sell products or services on the show and maybe even split the revenues to pay for air time. Or, if you cannot or do not want to produce and star in your own show, position yourself as an expert so you appear on other people's shows.

Follow this same advice for a radio show. Be a guest on as many talk shows as you can. If you have your own show, and you can do this by purchasing the time from the station, make certain you have listeners call in. Also, remember to mention your products and services, and give the listeners ways they can get in touch with you.

Brochures

Brochures are an excellent way to advertise your fitness business. Don't fall into the trap, however, of writing your own brochure. Experience has shown that technical professionals are experts in their field. When they write a brochure, they tend to write it as a technical or informational report. Your brochure must be a sales piece, and it must constantly sell for you when you are not there.

Invest some time and money and find professional marketing experts to help you with your brochure. Let these consultants hire the artists and printers and writers, and let them turn your concepts into tangible realities. Then, you can attend to the business of running your club while they create your masterpiece.

While the intricacies of developing a brochure are beyond the scope of this book, there are certain items you must consider: 1. Who is your audience? 2. What are you trying to sell them? 3. What methods will best communicate your message to them? 4. What type of budget is available to produce the brochure? 5. Will the brochure be black and white, one, two, three or four colors, and will it have pictures and/or illustrations? 6. How will the brochure be used: as a handout, a mailer, or a leave behind? 7. Will having the brochure help or hurt my business?

After you answer these 7 questions, you are ready to begin working on your brochure.

Flyers

Flyers are one page brochures, and they are also known as data sheets. Flyers are usually produced to announce openings, special events, programs, and unique classes. Make sure your flyer sells what you are selling. Use graphics, pictures, attention-getting phrases, and a call to action on every flyer.

Flyers can also be printed in multiple colors. This costs money, and you can achieve a similar effect just by using colored paper. Gold, royal blue, and some of the neon colors definitely attract attention, even when the flyer is printed in black ink.

Be original, creative, and innovative with your flyers. Code them as you would any other advertisement so you can track their effectiveness. You may be pleasantly surprised at the results these flyers bring.

Electronic Media

There is a proliferation of on-line computer bulletin boards. Find one that you can become a member of, let the other people know who you are and what you do, and then find out if you can advertise on the board. You may be surprised to learn that people have started successful businesses just by using on-line services.

Electronic billboards are another advertising method you can use. These flashing messages change every minute or so, and yours is placed in a rotation. This is different from a standard outdoor billboard where your message stays fixed for the contracted period of time. However, the electronic billboard does capture people's attention, especially motorists who are either passing by or stuck at a traffic light. You may want to check into these costs as an alternative advertising method.

Direct Response Advertising

This is more a repetition of my previous recommendation than anything else. You have probably already figured out that all advertising should be direct response advertising. By this, I mean that every communication message you send should tell the reader, listener or viewer to call, write or come in for more information or to do something else. You must motivate them to action.

Any advertising that is not direct response is just a waste of time, money and space. Remember, image advertising never put money in the bank. Only selling will do that, and you must use your advertising as salesmanship in print.

Promotions

Promotions are not advertising techniques in the way most people think of advertising. However, the purpose of a promotion is to stimulate business, make more people buy what you are selling, whether it is memberships or fitness programs, and to create attention for your business. Here are 10 types of promotions that you can consider using to stimulate business and support your marketing program. If you can think of more, by all means, use them.

1. Sampling - free giveaways of your products or services
2. Discounts - lower your prices for a specified time
3. Specialty items - key chains, calendars, bags, etc.
4. Contests - there must be a winner
5. Premiums - specialty items to expand your business, usually used as gifts with a purchase
6. Seminars and speeches - talk to your prospects and customers
7. Stamp plans - get enough stamps, get something for free
8. Coupons - two for one, discounts, or anything else
9. Exhibitions - show the public what you've got
10. Referral building - member get a member programs

Getting the Business to Come to You

Here are some final thoughts about advertising. Some of these are merely summaries of what has already been said in this chapter, and others provide new ideas or expand old ones. Consider each recommendation and how it will help business come to you, and then use it as is or adapt it accordingly to make your advertising twice as effective at half the price.

1. All advertising must be direct response. If they don't respond, how will you be able to track the ad's effectiveness?
2. Code all ads so you can track them.
3. All ads, regardless of their type, must have a headline that screams a benefit and arouses interest.
4. Subheads and body copy must always support the headline. In fact, write your copy first and then check it. Your best headline may be in one of the first four sentences.
5. Create all advertising from the customer's perspective. Don't create "me too" ads telling how great you are. Find out what your customers need and want, and then tell them in your ads how you will give it to them better than anyone else can.
6. Create all advertising using a features, advantages, benefits chart. Most people know a great deal about their features, but have a difficult time turning these features into advantages and benefits. For each feature of your product or service, describe why it is advantageous for a customer to do business with you or your club or facility and what benefits they will receive from this relationship.
7. Advertising must support the overall marketing plan. If the marketing plan is bad, no advertising in the world will save it. You will just be wasting money. Unless, of course, you have unlimited funds and can keep advertising in hopes of generating business.
8. Don't do image advertising. It is too expensive and it does not sell anything. If it doesn't sell, it doesn't generate revenue.

9. Consider the psychology of selling and advertising. Your customers have certain fears that you can help them put aside, and they have specific problems you can help them solve. When your ads address these fears and problems, and offer resolutions, you will find more people doing business with you.

10. Whatever you promise in your ads, make certain you can deliver on it. Never over promise and under deliver. It is always better to under promise and over deliver. In fact, this is one of the main principles for successful customer service.

11. If you advertise guarantees, make sure you can live up to them. Whether it is money back, free replacements, or anything else, live up to your guarantee as you advertise it.

12. Be creative, innovative and off the wall. You don't have to do everything the way your competitors do it. Find a way to make yourself stand out from the crowd.

13. Stay away from large ad agencies. Find individual consultants and freelancers to help you create your marketing programs and ad campaigns. The results will be just as good, the quality of the work will be just as high, and you will receive a great deal of personal attention.

14. Never advertise to replace a face to face contact. People buy from people, not from or because of ads. If you can sell to someone personally, do that. Don't substitute advertising for direct contact.

15. Give your ad campaigns a chance to work. If the advertising program is designed to support the marketing program, don't pull the ads after one or two placements. Give the ads a chance to be recognized and to work.

There you have it. A few suggestions on how to make your advertising twice as effective, and how to get twice the advertising at half the price. You will find many more suggestions in the chapter on free and inexpensive, yet effective marketing tactics. Remember to develop your advertising plan from the marketing plan, set the plan in motion and give it a chance to work, and then track its effectiveness. If, after a certain amount of time, you are not seeing the results you expected or desired, then it is time to change the advertising program. Check your research, your target markets, your messages, and everything else you were using to communicate with prospects and customers. Then revise the ads, implement the new ones, and give the new campaign a chance to work.

You want your advertising to generate business for you as soon as possible. If it cannot do this immediately, your advertising should at least generate interest in your business. Once the interest is there, it is up to you and your staff to convert the interested prospects into customers and members.

One last thought. Be consistent in your advertising messages. Don't jump around with slogans, pitches, and phrases. The more consistent you are, the more people will come to recognize your business and what you stand for. As an example, if you provide personal training for free, where every other facility charges for it, or a personal guarantee of satisfaction, have your ads state that personal training is free and the customer's satisfaction is guaranteed. Continuity and consistency of your messages will help to make your advertising twice as effective.

Creating Successful Customer Service

Chapter 7

Beyond Customer Service

Customer service is the buzzword of doing business in the 90's. You cannot hope to succeed in today's competitive fitness environment unless you can provide customer service that is far superior to that provided by your competitors.

Customer service does not only mean offering high quality programs, although program quality is an important part of customer service. After all, if someone buys a membership from or takes part in a program provided by you that is of poor quality, as the customer defines it, the odds are they will go somewhere else to get the programs and services they want. So, you must first provide customers with quality programs and services to win them over. Then, you must provide superior customer service to keep them, preferably for life.

Customer service involves all the activities your business and your employees conduct or perform to satisfy customers. This means more than just handling complaints, providing membership or purchase refunds or exchanges on returns, and smiling at customers. Customer service also means going out of your way for the member/customer, doing everything possible to satisfy the customer, and making decisions that benefit the customer even at the expense of your club, wellness center, or company.

Now, I am not saying that you should give away the store to the member or customer. I am saying that you have to know when and how often the customer is always right. Then, you make your decisions based on the situation, what the customer wants, and how it affects your facility.

The Importance of Customer Service

Customer service does not cost, IT PAYS. It pays in a variety of ways, the first of which is long-term customer or member retention. Some fitness businesses are aware of the cost of acquiring a new customer, while others do not have a clue what new member acquisition costs them. Furthermore, most fitness professionals are also not aware of the extraordinary costs of losing a member/customer. In fact, you should know that it costs 5 to 6 times more to acquire a new customer than it does to do business with a current or former customer (member). Add to this the costs of replacing lost customers and you have a great deal of money that could have dropped to the bottom line.

This is important because the fitness industry is such a low profit margin business. The more money that drops to the bottom line, the more profitable you will be. Customer service and satisfaction, along with long-term retention, are vitally important to your success in this industry.

I am sure you realize that high quality customer service is both a marketing and a management tool for your business. It enhances marketing because it motivates customers to spread the word about your service and business to others, creating, in effect, a member/customer sales force. Remember, the least expensive way to acquire new members/customers is through word of mouth referrals. Good service improves management because everybody is committed to satisfying the customer. The results are increased productivity and profits simply because management and employees are working to achieve the same goal: customer satisfaction and retention.

In order to achieve this goal, you must develop a customer service system for your club, company or facility. This system must be easily accessible by the customers and easy for them to use. The next thing you must do is design and implement proactive customer retention programs. These activities are designed to maintain customer loyalty and to motivate them to maintain their membership with you, make ongoing purchases from you, and provide you with a steady stream of referrals.

Here is a simple 7-step system for developing a successful customer service program.

7 Steps to Developing a Successful Customer Service System

Step 1. Total Management Commitment
Customer service programs and member retention programs cannot succeed unless senior management is totally committed to the concept. It is up to the president, CEO or owner to develop a clear and concise **service vision** for the company. Then, management must communicate that vision to all the employees, members and program participants. The vision and the commitment can be verbalized as part of the company's service mission statement.

If you do not have a corporate mission statement, and/or a service mission statement, you should develop them right now, and post them in a highly visible and conspicuous place for everyone to see your total commitment to 100% customer satisfaction.

Step 2. Get to Know Your Customers
Successful member retention and customer service programs require that you know your customers intimately and understand them totally. You need to know what they like about you, your staff and your facility and programs, what they dislike, what they want changed, how they want it changed, what needs they have, what their expectations are, what motivates them to buy from you, what satisfies them, and what you must continue to do to maintain their loyalty to you over time. The most effective way to do this is simply to ask your customers to provide you with this information.

Once you start to know your customers, you must keep on learning about them. Their needs change on a regular, and even daily basis. You must keep up with them. Make it a policy to call your member/customers at least once a month to find out how they are doing and what they need. Invite them to meet with you as an advisory group to make recommendations to help you improve your service. This shows them you are interested in providing good customer service, and it also helps you develop effective customer retention programs.

Step 3. Develop Standards of Service Quality Performance

Many people think it is difficult to develop measurable standards of service quality performance, because service is an intangible and intangibles are hard to measure. However, there are ways to develop these performance standards, and you must make them specific to your fitness business. When you have developed these standards, you will begin to see superior performance by your employees. Remember, **what gets measured gets done**. Usually, when people just know that their customer service performance is going to be measured, their service to customers improves.

Step 4. Hire, Train and Compensate Superior Staff

Good customer service and effective customer/member retention programs can only be provided by competent, qualified and well-trained people. Your service is only as good as the people who deliver it. If you want your business to be nice to people, hire nice people.

Then, train them to provide the ultimate in customer service and retention programs. Pay them well as they are the primary reason people will continue to do business with you. Also, give them the authority to make decisions on the spot to satisfy customers, even if they sometimes have to bend the company rules and regulations.

Remember that serving and retaining customers is one of the hardest jobs in a company. If people have that responsibility, they must also have the authority to decide what they can and cannot do for a customer. Give them that authority, and you will see your customer retention efforts improve dramatically.

Step 5. Reward Service Accomplishments

You must always reward and reinforce superior performances. Provide financial and psychological rewards and incentives for your staff. Recognize and praise the small wins and accomplishments the same way you would applaud and dramatize the major wins. Always remember that **what gets rewarded gets done**.

You must also reward your members/customers for good customer behavior. They appreciate recognition the same way your employees do. Recognizing your member/customers will go a long way towards retaining them and having them refer new people to you.

Step 6. Stay Close to Your Customers

Maintain constant contact with your customers. Conduct continuous and ongoing research to learn from them. Ask them questions right after they join, take a class, work out, make a purchase, or do anything with your club or facility that allows them to form an opinion. Send them surveys in the mail, run contests that require participation in a survey, hold focus groups to get perceptions and opinions of your fitness business, call them on the telephone, develop a customer council to advise you on their needs, and do anything else you must do to stay close to your customers.

Be aware that your relationship with the member/customer actually began before the purchase was made. This is when you must activate your retention programs, and this is when the customer will get to see how much you really care. Arrange all customer interactions so they are win-win situations for both of you. The result will be more loyal customers and longer term members.

Step 7. Work Towards Continuous Improvement

Even though you have designed easy to use, friendly, and easily accessible customer service systems, you have hired and trained the best staff possible, and you go out of your way to learn about and satisfy your customers needs, you must remember that no system, business or program is perfect. Therefore, you must work to continuously improve your customer service programs and your retention activities.

Your attempts at continuous improvement will be viewed very positively by member/ customers and employees. They will see this as an attempt to become even better than you already are. The results of continuously improving your customer service systems and programs are more satisfied customers, more business for you and your staff, and greater profits.

These are the 7 basic steps you need to follow to develop an effective customer service system. As I said before, customer service pays, it does not cost. You must constantly work to provide the best service at all times. Your only goal for being in the fitness business, or any business for that matter, should be to satisfy your customers. Once this is done, the growth, expansion and profits will take care of themselves. Follow these 7 steps and you will find that it will be very easy for you to go beyond customer service to long-term member/ customer retention.

An Example of Quality Customer Service

Here is a very common example of how to provide quality customer service that goes beyond the rules and regulations, policies and procedures, and contracts associated with joining a club or a wellness center. We all know that you usually allow people a 72 hour "cooling off" period after they sign a membership contract and pay a deposit or the full amount to join.

Now, this new member decides to withdraw his or her membership, but it is one week later. Obviously, it is past the "cooling off" period. The new member does not have any valid medical reason for wanting his or her money back. What do you do? YOU GIVE IT BACK WITH NO QUESTIONS ASKED. Then, you offer them a two week FREE membership to continue working out and participating in your programs. You may never get them as a member, but you certainly went **beyond customer service** to show them how much you really care.

The next thing this "lost" member/customer will do is tell up to five friends or colleagues about the terrific service you provided. They will be so happy to receive their money back, they will think that you are the greatest service provider in the world. Now, isn't this much better than having them not receive their money back and tell up to 20 of their friends what type of terrible service you provide?

Here are 10 other reasons you should go out of your way to bend your policies and give this person their money back. These are what I call startling service statistics, and they are compiled from a variety of sources.

Startling Service Statistics

1. Only 4% of customers ever complain. That means your fitness business may never hear from 96% of its customers or members, and 91% of those people just go away because they feel complaining will not do them any good. In fact, complainers are more likely to continue doing business with you than non-complainers.

2. For every complaint you receive, there are 26 other customers with unresolved complaints or problems, and 6 of those people have serious problems. These are people you probably will never hear from. These are also people with answers as to how you can make your business better. Get their feedback any way you can, even if you have to beg for it.

3. Between 54% and 70% of customers who complain to you will do business with you again if you resolve their complaint. If they feel you acted quickly and to their satisfaction, then up to 95% of them will do business with you again, and they probably will refer other people to you.

4. A dissatisfied customer or member will tell up to 10 people about their dissatisfaction. Approximately 13% of those will tell up to 20 people about their problem. You cannot afford the advertising to overcome this negative word of mouth, especially since people tend to embellish and over-exaggerate their stories as the time gets further away from the actual event.

5. Happy customers, or customers who have had their problems or complaints resolved, will tell between 3 and 5 people about their positive experience. Therefore, you have to satisfy 3 to 4 customers or members for every one that is dissatisfied with you. It is very difficult in any business to work with a 4:1 ratio against you. This fact becomes even more important because the fitness business is such a low margin industry. Now you know why customer satisfaction and customer retention programs help and enhance the value of your customer service efforts.

6. It costs 5 to 6 times more to attract new customers than to keep old ones, even when you have to go back and renew contacts with former customers and contracts with former members. Additionally, customer loyalty and the lifetime value of a customer can be worth up to 10 times as much as the price of a single purchase. Remember that next time you are trying to make some quick membership sales just to boost revenue in a particular month.

7. Fitness businesses that provide superior customer service can charge more, realize greater profits, increase their market share, and have customers or members willingly pay more for their products and services simply because of the good service. In fact, you can gain an average of 6% a year in market share simply by providing good service, satisfying and keeping your customers.

8, The lifetime value of a customer, or the amount of purchases that a customer would make over a 10 year period, is worth more than the cost of returning their purchase price of one item. For example, supermarkets realize up to $5,000 a year from one family. That means $50,000 over 10 years. Is it worth it for them to provide refunds when the customer returns a purchase? Is it worth it to you to have the good will and positive word of mouth this type of retention service will bring you? Think back to the previous example of returning a membership fee after the "cooling off" period has expired. Is it worth it now in light of all these statistics related to customer service and satisfaction?

9. Customer service is governed by the rules of 10's. If it costs $10,000 to get a new customer, it takes only 10 seconds to lose one, and 10 years to get over it or for the problem to finally be resolved. You must work to keep your customers.

10. Customers stop doing business with you because:
    - 1% die
    - 3% move away
    - 5% seek alternatives or develop other business relationships
    - 9% begin doing business with the competition
    - 14% are dissatisfied with the product or service
    - 68% are upset with the treatment they have received

Despite these startling service statistics, there is good news. And that is you have control over 96% of the reasons people stop doing business with you. Furthermore, over 80% of the reasons people stop doing business with a company are related to service quality and performance issues rather than product quality or product performance. Do you see why customer service, retention and satisfaction are so important to the success of your fitness business? Do you also understand why providing superior service, retention and satisfaction programs are essential to your marketing efforts?

NOW, WHAT WILL YOU DO SO YOU DO NOT BECOME ONE OF THESE STARTLING SERVICE STATISTICS?

Customers and club members today are better educated than ever before. They are more careful about their purchases and the dollars they spend. They are tired of constantly receiving poor service. They want value for their money, especially since fitness purchases and club memberships are perceived as discretionary income. They also want good service, and they are willing to pay for it. Quite simply, customers expect more for their purchases, and if they get it, they will pay for it. Therefore, it is only through customer service and retention programs that you will be able to maintain your market share, competitive edge, keep your current customers, and remain profitable to stay in business.

Reasons For Poor Service

Ask any consumer, former club member, or for that matter, ask yourself, why companies give such poor service. You will receive a whole host of reasons. Some of them may be unique to the fitness industry while others tend to be more global. Here are 10 of the more "popular" reasons for giving or receiving poor customer service. How many of them apply to your fitness business or organization?

- Uncaring employees
- Poorly trained employees
- Differences in perceptions between what fitness directors think customers/members want and what customers actually want
- Differences in perceptions between what fitness directors or business owners think they provide customers in the way of service and what customers actually receive, or perceive they receive
- No customer service philosophy within the fitness company
- Employees are not empowered to provide good service, take responsibility and make decisions that will satisfy the customer.
- Negative attitudes of employees toward customers (sometimes this is due to the negative attitudes of management toward its employees or just the way management treats its employees)
- Differences in perceptions between the way fitness directors think customers want to be treated and the way customers really want to be treated
- Poor handling and resolution of complaints
- Poor treatment of employees as customers

Add your own reasons to this list of 10, then do one more thing. Develop a system for measuring your customer service and level of customer satisfaction. When you have this information, you will begin to realize why it is imperative to not only provide superior customer service, but to go beyond customer service and do everything possible to acquire, maintain and retain loyal customers and members.

One more point must be made about customer loyalty before moving on to how you actually retain customers. People are loyal to your fitness facility because they feel they are treated well, they receive good value for their money, and they are psychologically or physically attached to the club or business somehow. You must do everything possible to make certain that your customers/members do not want to switch to your competitors.

NEVER TAKE A CUSTOMER FOR GRANTED. BE GRATEFUL THEY HAVE DECIDED TO DO BUSINESS WITH YOU AND NOT A COMPETITOR. WORK AS HARD AS YOU POSSIBLY CAN TO DELIVER MORE THAN THEY EXPECT, AND YOU WILL HAVE GONE A LONG WAY TOWARD SERVICING, RETAINING AND SATISFYING YOUR CUSTOMERS.

Customer Service as a Marketing Tactic

Now that you are keenly aware of the importance of customer service, how to set up your customer service program and use it to satisfy and retain customers/members, you are ready to use a variety of service techniques as marketing strategies and tactics. This section describes a wide variety of tools and you can use to go beyond customer service, increase customer retention, and enhance your marketing efforts all at the same time. These 7 service/marketing techniques will help your fitness business grow and become more profitable, regardless of competition or economic conditions.

Frequent Buyer Program

Frequent buyer programs are similar to the airlines' frequent flyer programs. You are rewarding those customers or members who buy from you on a regular basis. Regular buying can mean memberships for family and friends, products, programs, or ongoing services. You must define what they are buying and how frequently they must buy in order to be rewarded.

The rewards do not have to be expensive or lavish. They just have to show the customer you appreciate their business. Also, it should not be difficult for your regular customers to benefit from this program.

Consider a fitness center that punches a card every time a member brings a guest. After your tenth or twelfth guest, the club gives that member something for free, or at a significant discount: a 1-hour personal training session or a workout bag. The club is encouraging the member to continue to bring guests because then the club can turn the guests into members. This way, everyone wins. The club gets more revenue, the member gets rewarded for positive behaviors (which are then reinforced and become very likely to occur again), and the guests win because they get to use the club and possibly join for their own enjoyment.

Frequent buyer programs are an excellent way to retain customers and keep them coming back for more.

Frequent Referral Programs

These are similar to the frequent buyer programs. Since your fitness business depends on referrals, you should reward the people making referrals to you. Your rewards will also reinforce their behavior, thereby creating a positive cycle and a mutually beneficial relationship.

The best way to use a frequent referral reward program is to develop it in tiers, or levels. This means that the referral source will receive certain rewards from you based on the number of referrals. For example, you may simply send the person a thank you card for the first referral. The second referral warrants a telephone call with another card. The third referral receives a small, inexpensive gift that has some perceived value. The fourth referral may receive a free membership or a free program registration. The fifth referral definitely should be rewarded with a dinner gift certificate to a very nice restaurant. Then, you can start the entire process all over again.

Use these suggestions or develop some of your own. The important thing is to reward the people who refer new customers/members to you. This reinforces their behavior, makes them feel good, and they will continue to refer because you acknowledged their efforts.

Here is another suggestion, but before you use it, make certain your referral sources do not mind having their name visible in your club or office. Create a Referral Thank You Bulletin Board. Put all the names of your current members/customers who refer new members/customers to you on this board each month. You can also put the number of referrals they have made. People usually like to see their name written on something, and this will give them the satisfaction of knowing you appreciate their efforts.

You can also take this a step further. Create a New Customer Welcome Bulletin Board. List all the names of your new customers/members each month. This is the first step in a proactive customer retention program. When new members or customers see that you care enough to put their names up for everyone else to see, they will go out of their way to help you make your fitness business successful.

Thank You Cards

This is one of the simplest and most effective customer service and retention techniques, yet not enough fitness businesses send them out. It only takes a little bit of extra effort on your part to write out a card and address an envelope and send it to someone who has done business with you (joined your facility, registered for a program, or bought something from you). It is the best postage stamp marketing investment you can make.

You can either write out a thank you card every time you need to send one, or you can have your cards pre-printed with a message that shows your appreciation. It is even more effective if you develop part of your customer service and retention program around a series of these cards.

Here are some samples of pre-printed cards that I use for all my customers. You can make them up at your local printer or purchase them from a specialty dealer. The cards are sent out in the order you see them: 1) Thank you for your business; 2) Our customers are number 1; and when the job is completed, 3) It was a pleasure to serve you. When my company receives a referral, we send out the referral thank you card. All this information and the dates the cards are sent are tracked through our customer database.

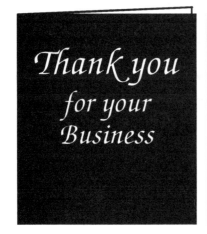

| Inside: Your business is greatly appreciated. | Inside: We appreciate the opportunity to serve you! | Inside: We were very glad to serve you and we look forward to having the same opportunity again! |

You can also include holiday and birthday cards in this card marketing program. Your customers/members will appreciate receiving these from you. They will know that it is another way for you to show you care about them.

Newsletters

Newsletters are an excellent way to keep your customers and members informed of what is going on in your fitness business. You can provide them with whatever information you need them to know. And, because it is coming from you free of charge, they will most probably read every word of it.

One way to keep your customers involved with your business is to promote contests or other activities in the newsletter. Then, make it so they have to come to your club or office to "win" the contest. When they arrive, make every effort to solidify their loyalty and retain them as customers. If it is a prospect who has come to see you, do everything you can from a service perspective to convert this person to a customer or member.

Here is a great variation of the newsletter I mentioned earlier. It is called a letter of news. You write a personal letter to each customer (using a computerized customer database makes this task very easy) and mention all the items you would have mentioned in a newsletter. Just use sub-headings in this personal letter as you would article headings in the newsletter. Also, feel free to bold your subheadings or important pieces of information. Your customers will be very pleased that you took the time to write them a personal letter and they probably will read every word of it, especially if you keep it to one or two pages.

Telephone Recalls

Telephone recalls work very well in all aspects of the fitness industry where appointments are necessary, such as private training or classes, meetings, fitness testing, nutritional counseling, or anything else that may require a reminder as a nice touch of service. All you do is call them a day in advance to remind them of the appointment. Or, if they have not been in to see you in quite some time, you can call them up to see how they are doing and to inform them of a reason to come in now to do business with you (new classes, programs, equipment and services are all valid reasons to call).

Here are four customer service hints to prevent telephone abuse. 1. When the customer answers your telephone call, or you answer an incoming call, always give your name and the name of your company. 2. Never put a caller on hold for more than 30 seconds without first asking permission to place them on hold, and then coming back to them to tell them how much longer you will be. 3. If your customers are complaining they are having trouble getting through to you on the telephone, it may be time to install more telephone lines or numbers. You may even want to consider an 800 number, since the rates are now very respectable for small business *(see Fitness)* owners. 4. Try not to call people at dinner time or too late in the evening.

Reward and Recognition Programs

This is really very simple. Positive reinforcement motivates people to engage in the same behavior that was rewarded again and again. Figure out what types of rewards you want to offer employees, members and customers, decide on how you will recognize their efforts on your behalf, and then just do it. Your reward and recognition programs will be even more effective if they come at unexpected times.

Unexpected rewards or recognition are among the most powerful motivators and reinforcers of human behavior. Also, you need to acknowledge and reward the small accomplishments just as you do the major wins. Everybody likes to have their ego stroked. The better you do this, the more profitable you will be since people will tell other people to come to your club, participate in your classes or programs, or just buy products from you.

Walk Your Talk

Get out and be seen by your staff and your members/customers. Be a role model of excellent service. Do whatever it takes to service, satisfy and retain your members/customers. Act the same way towards your staff. They will, in turn, treat the members/customers the same way you do.

Many fitness directors, club owners and entrepreneurs say they provide excellent service. While that may be true, not enough people are using their service as a marketing strategy. Your visibility is critical to the success of your service/marketing program. Use customer service as a marketing tool, then go beyond customer service to achieve customer satisfaction. The only way you will know if you are satisfying your customers is to ask them.

Measuring Customer Satisfaction

Customer satisfaction measurement seems to be the step child of marketing and customer service in the fitness industry. While there are facilities that take some measurements, many of these facilities don't know what to do with their information. One club I worked with handed out written member satisfaction surveys every quarter. They got the surveys back, read them over, and then filed them. When I asked the director what was done with the information, she told me "I don't know. I guess the owners do something with it". Now that's scary.

Measure everything that you want to have done and improved. Remember, what gets measured gets done, so if you want to service your customers and make sure they are satisfied, measure your efforts. Then, score the surveys or the interviews so you have quantifiable information. Next, share the information with your staff members. They will provide better service if they know what areas need to be improved.

Oh, by the way, I met with the owners and taught them how to score and use survey data to improve their service, member retention and profitability. That was in 1990. In 1992, their member satisfaction ratings have gone from 65% overall to 97%. It really was very simple. The surveys told the owners exactly what the customers liked and disliked. All they had to do was implement some of the recommended changes. Once this was done, the members were more satisfied, they referred more people, and the staff improved their service levels.

Don't Forget the Quality

When we think of service in the fitness industry, or in any business, we also must think of quality. We talk about quality facilities, quality programs, quality equipment, a high quality staff, and the like. Don't just talk about it. DO IT!!

Work every day to measure and improve your quality. Don't try to do one thing 1000% better. Do 1000 things 1% better every day. For example, if all your aerobics instructors worked to improve their classes by 1/2% every day, their classes would be about 25% better by the end of the year. The same numbers hold true for all your operating systems.

Improving quality is not a one time thing. It is an ongoing process of never-ending improvement. It begins with a commitment by management or owners, a new philosophy of doing business, and a whole new attitude towards employees and customers. The next chapter gives you 50 ways you can improve your quality, customer service, levels of customer satisfaction, and retention.

Keeping Customers

Chapter 8

50 Ways to Keep Your Customers For Life

This book has given you numerous ideas and methods that you can use to market, service, satisfy and retain your members/customers. Additionally, this book has provided you with methods to go beyond customer service and use your service efforts as additional ways to market your fitness facility or program more effectively. Now, here is a list of 50 things (tips, tricks, techniques, methods, strategies and tactics) you can use to service, satisfy and retain your customers and members.

1. CREATE A SERVICE ORIENTED CULTURE - Everyone in the company must be customer service oriented. All employees must realize that they work for the customer, and their job is to ensure the ultimate satisfaction of the customer or member. Everything else really doesn't matter because without members, you have no fitness business.

2. HAVE A SERVICE VISION - A service vision is vital to the success of any organization. This vision must be more than just a philosophy of doing business. It must be the corporate cultural ethic. Everyone must believe and live the vision in order for your fitness company to provide excellent customer service and keep customers for life.

3. TOTAL SUPPORT - Many books recommend having top management support for a customer service and retention program. True success comes from having total support throughout the organization. Remember, while it may be top management who decides to embark on a customer service or member retention program, it is the employees who actually implement the program. If these people do not support the service initiative, then the program will not work. Remember that total support is needed.

4. POLICIES IN WRITING - Put your service policies in writing. This is as much for the benefit of the customers as it is for your employees. This way, there can be no mistakes or misunderstandings. Just be aware, though, that there will be exceptions to your policies and your employees have to be able to deal with those exceptions at the time they occur.

5. EMPLOYEE EMPOWERMENT - Give your employees the authority to go with their tremendous responsibility of satisfying and keeping the customer. Allow them to make decisions on the spot that will benefit both the club and the member. Then, you support those decisions. Remember, their job is to satisfy the customers/members and to keep them coming back. Employees should not have to look for you every time a member/ customer needs something out of the ordinary.

6. EMPLOYEE TRAINING - Train, train, and then re-train to retain your employees. Give them on the job training, off the job training, tapes, books, seminars, workshops, anything, that will help them do their jobs better. While you may find qualified people who have just graduated school, nothing prepares a person better for dealing with customers and serving and satisfying members than the training they receive on the job and in applied programs.

7. MARKETING THE SERVICE PROGRAM - All of your marketing efforts must communicate your service message, that you are interested only in total customer satisfaction, and that you will do everything possible to keep your customers. This message must be stated in every ad, commercial, flyer, brochure and press release you send out to the public and to the trades.

8. HIRE GOOD PEOPLE - This means hiring people who are good and nice in addition to their being well qualified. People who are nice to other people are usually nice people themselves. These innate people skills will go a long way toward helping your staff provide superior customer service and retain your customers. This is even more important in the fitness industry because it is such an intense people industry. If there ever was a business that was dependent on "high touch", fitness is it. Good and nice people will help you succeed.

9. DON'T MAKE CUSTOMERS PAY FOR SERVICE - You should be willing to pay for anything related to customer service. This includes shipping charges when they return a product to you, long distance telephone calls, return postage, and anything else the customer would normally pay in order to receive service from you. If you do not pay for the cost of service, your competition will. And then, your customers/members will become their customers/members.

10. REWARD LOYALTY - What gets rewarded gets done. Reward loyalty on the part of both your customers and your employees. Do this, and they both will stay with you a long time. Remember, the rewards have to be perceived as valuable by the recipient. In reality, they actually do not have to be expensive.

11. INSPECT WHAT YOU EXPECT - What gets measured gets done. Measure the performance of your staff members and you will see an increase in performance levels, quality and productivity. Also, measure the quality of their service. Finally, measure the satisfaction levels of your customers and members.

12. SET STANDARDS OF PERFORMANCE - Let everyone know exactly what they must do to provide superior customer service. Make these standards as objective and measurable as possible, even though you are dealing with an intangible service. When your staff achieves these performance levels, customer retention and loyalty naturally follow.

13. TRADE JOBS - Have your employees experience working in other departments. You should also trade jobs with all your employees. This way, everyone will develop an

appreciation for what other people in the facility or company do. The result is that no employee will blame another one for a customer problem. In fact, since the employees have experience in other areas, they will be able to solve more problems and satisfy more customers on the spot.

14. CROSS TRAIN - THIS IS AN EXTENSION OF #13. Train your employees in other people's jobs. This enables them to provide more assistance to customers. It also helps you from becoming too dependent on one employee who seems irreplaceable because no one else can do his or her job. Furthermore, cross training promotes the development of a team philosophy of cooperation, instead of a "we-they" competitive philosophy. This attitude will be communicated to and appreciated by your customers/ members.

15. EASILY ACCESSIBLE SERVICE SYSTEMS - Make your service systems easy for the customer to access. Have them reach a person on the telephone as soon as they call the club or office, or have them speak with an employee who can help them as soon as they arrive at your club. If they have a complaint, go to them if you must and do everything in your power to resolve it. Don't make it hard for customers to come to you. They will perceive this as negative and then decide not to do business with you again.

16. USER FRIENDLY SERVICES SYSTEMS - Make your customer service systems user friendly, meaning easy for them to use. The member/customer is the reason for your business, not someone who is in the way of doing business. Make them feel and know they can bring a problem to your attention, voice a complaint and get it resolved as quickly as possible, and receive superb treatment during all their contacts with your company.

17. DESIGN FLEXIBILITY INTO YOUR SERVICE POLICIES - Policies were mentioned earlier as being important. You must have flexible and adaptable policies because each customer and each situation is different. Your employees must know they can modify a written or stated policy to ensure the customer's total satisfaction at any given moment. This means taking a little extra time and making a little extra effort to treat everyone as an individual, and it is well worth it.

18. EDUCATE THE CUSTOMER - You should not assume anything on the part of the member/customer. Use every customer contact as a chance to educate the customer about something related to your business. Even if you are just educating them about your great renewal policy, teach them. They will be appreciative and show this by continuing to do business with you.

19. HANDLE COMPLAINTS PROPERLY - Here is the simplest and most effective method for handling complaints. Acknowledge the customer is upset, listen carefully, assure them you are doing everything possible at this moment to resolve their complaint, and then resolve the complaint. Then, when they are appreciative of your efforts, use the opportunity to increase their loyalty. Thank them for bringing the

problem to your attention, apologize again for the problem, and maybe even try to sell them something else.

19. TURN COMPLAINTS INTO ADDITIONAL SALES - After you resolve a complaint, the customer is most receptive to continuing to do business with you. This is a good time, and it is definitely ethical, to try to sell them something else. In fact, they will be appreciative of your interest in them. They will probably buy from you now, and go out and tell their friends how well and how quickly you handled their problem. You will develop the reputation with customers of being credible, reliable and trustworthy.

20. TRAIN YOUR EMPLOYEES TO DO IT RIGHT THE FIRST TIME - This will save you money plus make customers very happy that they do not have to return anything or complain. Repair, rework or additional free services are very costly. Doing it right the first time guarantees greater profitability, happier customers and more long term customers. This is the essence of quality service.

21. EVERY CUSTOMER HAS A LIFE TIME VALUE (LTV) - When a customer buys from you, whether it is a product or a membership, remember that it is not a one time, one price purchase. Consider the potential that person brings to your fitness business. How much money could that person spend with you over a lifetime? That amount is the lifetime value of a customer and that is the type of service they should receive *every* time they do business with you.

If their LTV is $5000.00, then they should receive $5000.00 worth of service every time they come to your club, a class, a program, or an event. Go beyond expected customer service performance and show the people that you appreciate them and respect their potential lifetime value to your fitness business.

22. ASK, DEMAND, EVEN BEG FOR CUSTOMER FEEDBACK - It is not just enough to send out surveys or leave comment cards at the front desk. You must get as much customer feedback as possible, even if you have to beg for it. When members/ customers are asked their opinion, and then they see you have implemented their suggestions, they will not only continue to do business with you, they will recommend that friends come to you also. Do whatever you can to solicit their opinions and comments, and then act on their recommendations.

23. IDENTIFY CUSTOMER VALUES, BELIEFS AND STANDARDS - Your service programs must be geared to the values, beliefs and standards of your members/ customers. This will tell them you are interested in them and they will want to stay with you for longer periods of time. Set up all your service programs so they are geared to and for the customer rather than for your fitness business. If there is a conflict between customer values and your values, invite your members/customers into the facility for a discussion to find out why the difference exists and what can be done about it. Then, decide if you must modify your position to maintain customer satisfaction and loyalty.

24. GET AND USE EMPLOYEE IDEAS - Your employees have daily contact with members/customers. The employees know more about what members/customers

need, want and expect than you or any other manager could ever hope to know. Get feedback from your employees, listen carefully to their suggestions, and then implement as many of them as possible. Research shows that the best service companies not only get more ideas from their employees, they use more of them. This also makes employees feel wanted and cared about. Although there is not yet research to support this same position for the fitness industry, it seems logical and obvious that the same thing would hold true.

25. BE FAIR AND CONSISTENT - Members/customers may not always like or agree with what you are doing for them, but as long as you treat each one fairly and consistently, they will respect you for it. This also enhances your credibility, which is essential for building loyalty and retaining members/customers.

26. UNDER PROMISE AND OVER DELIVER - One of the ways fitness businesses fail to satisfy and keep their members/customers is that they over promise and under deliver. This sets up some very high expectations on the part of the customer. Often times, the club has difficulty reaching these expectations, and the customer goes away disappointed. On the other hand, if you set realistic expectations for the customer regarding your quality and level of service, and then you exceed those expectations, the customer is more than satisfied. Remember, though, that you should not under promise to such an extent that it is insulting to the members/customers. They will see through you in a minute and take their business elsewhere.

27. COMPETE ON BENEFITS, NOT PRODUCTS OR PRICES - Members/customers can always find another product, program or club at a lower price, somehow, somewhere. You must always remind your members/customers of the benefits of doing business with you. Features can be found in every product or program, but benefits are unique to the way you do business. Promote your benefits to the members/customers on a personal level and they will stay with you.

28. HIGH TOUCH IS MORE IMPORTANT THAN HIGH TECH - It is true that high tech gets people to say "WOW!", but it doesn't get people to care about other people. Your fitness business needs high touch in order to survive in this industry. Every club seems to have the latest in high tech equipment. Therefore, stay close to the customer. Get to know each other well. The closer you are to the customer, the longer they will do business with you. After all, when you show you care, you become like one of their family, and they become like one of yours.

29. ASK MEMBERS/CUSTOMERS WHAT THEY WANT - Constantly ask your members/ customers what they want from you, what you can do for them, and how you can do it better. They may want a new product or service, extended hours, or just something minor that will make them happier. You will never know unless you ask. After you ask, you must give them what they want. They will reward your generosity with loyalty, more referrals and higher satisfaction ratings.

30. DAILY SERVICE MANAGEMENT - Every employee in every department is involved in providing superior service with the ultimate goal being to keep the customer for life.

You should do everything possible to make everyone's job easier, and the employees should work together (think about team building) to make their jobs easier and to make it easy for the members/customers to get what they want. If there is a problem during the day, make the necessary adjustments and resolve it quickly. The goal of everyone on your staff is to satisfy and retain members/customers. Never forget that.

31. KNOW THE COST OF LOSING A CUSTOMER - All employees should know the lifetime value of a customer to your fitness business. They should also know the cost of losing even just one customer and the effect it can have on your business. You can be sure that employees who are paid on an incentive basis according to how many members/customers are retained over a certain time period will do every thing they can to service those members/customers, and to solicit referrals from them for new members/customers.

32. KNOW YOUR COMPETITION - What are your competitors providing in the way of customer service? What are they doing to retain their members/customers? Are they offering more benefits, better service policies, or are they just being nicer to their members/customers? Find out, and if they are doing something you are not doing, then just do it. If it works for them, it will probably work for you. If you need to adapt it, adapt it. You don't have to re-invent the wheel here. Just learn what your competitors are doing and do it better, faster and with a bigger smile (better service).

33. CONDUCT ONGOING MARKET RESEARCH - You can never have enough information about your members/customers. Do surveys, questionnaires, focus groups, interviews, whatever it takes to find out what the marketplace wants. Hold member advisory forums where you invite them into your business to tell you how to improve. Then, adapt your fitness business, its programs and services, accordingly. Information is not power unless you know how to use it.

34. CONDUCT INTERNAL ASSESSMENTS - Constantly evaluate what your company is doing in the area of customer service, satisfaction, and retention. Interview your employees, have them fill out questionnaires, ask your members/customers at the point of purchase (when they join, after a class, after a workout, etc.) how you are doing, and then use this information to improve your service and retention efforts. Also, you can use this information to enhance your overall marketing and sales programs.

35. KNOW WHAT YOUR MEMBERS/CUSTOMERS NEED, WANT AND EXPECT - Here is where all businesses run into problems, especially fitness businesses. Fitness directors and club owners think they know exactly what members/customers need, want or expect. In reality, you think one thing when the customers/members really require another. This causes gaps in perceptions about service delivery that ultimately lead to lost members/customers. Find out what the members/customers need, want and expect, then give it to them. Close those perceptual gaps so you can retain your members/customers.

36. FIND, NURTURE AND DISPLAY CUSTOMER CHAMPIONS - Every fitness business has one or two, or several, employees who are true customer champions. Find out who these people are, nurture and support them, then make them role models for everyone else to follow. Reward their behavior in a variety of ways. The rest of your staff will upgrade their service performance to this level in order to receive similar rewards. The result is a highly motivated, service-oriented staff and a group of satisfied and loyal members/customers. Furthermore, you will realize an increase in revenues and profitability.

37. EFFECTIVE COMMUNICATION IS CRITICAL TO SUCCESS - This is especially true in the customer service area. Every problem between people is the result of poor communication. Members/customers did not understand what you meant, you did not understand them, or there was simply confusion about a policy or an agreement. The best way to resolve this is through interpersonal communication. Therefore, train your people to develop effective communication skills: how to speak so others will listen, how to listen first, how to understand others before trying to be understood, how to receive and give feedback, and how to develop rapport with members/customers.

38. RAPPORT IS THE KEY TO SUCCESSFUL COMMUNICATION - The technical aspects of communication skills can be acquired and used, but if there is no rapport, there is no true communication. The skills of developing rapport can be taught, and your employees should learn them. When employees and members/customers are in rapport, there is a feeling of trust and a desire to continue to do business. When both these aspects are used, you will have excellent communications with a customer.

39. SMILE - Smiles are important when dealing with your members. Smiles will usually get a smile in return, but smiles will not guarantee quality customer service. Smile training is not service training. Smiles must be part of the employees' everyday character and behavior, and it must be something they do because it makes them feel good which, in turn, makes the members/customers feel good. The best way to get your employees to smile is to hire happy people for your fitness facility. Of course, make sure they are qualified.

40. MAKE MEMBERS/CUSTOMERS FEEL IMPORTANT - The more important you make members/customers feel, the more and longer they will do business with you. Teach yourself and your staff to view everyone as if they had a sign across their chest that read "Make Me Feel Important". Call them by name, ask them to tell you about themselves, their family members (especially children and grandchildren) and ask questions about their accomplishments. Do whatever it takes to make them feel important. Your reward will be a lifetime customer and a significant number of new referrals.

41. PROMOTE YOUR MEMBERS/CUSTOMERS - That's right, your members/customers. Use them in your marketing and promotion efforts, with their permission, of course. Let them tell their story to other members/customers and prospects. This third party endorsement provides you with tremendous credibility and your members/customers will enjoy helping you and being involved with your fitness business. An additional

benefit is that when you promote them in your marketing programs, they will promote you in the community as a natural response to your including them.

42. CREATE A CUSTOMER COUNCIL - This is like a board of directors, only made up of just your members/customers. It can also serve as a focus group. The purpose of this group is to meet regularly to scrutinize your fitness business and the service you are providing. The council makes suggestions and you act on those suggestions. Membership in the council makes members/customers feel like they are part of your fitness business, and this breeds loyalty and long term retention.

43. MARKET FREQUENT BUYER PROGRAMS - This is a reward program for your frequent buyers. You can use coupons, punch cards or anything else that helps you keep track of how often members/customers do business with you. The program can even be adapted to referrals. Then, when they reach a certain purchase level, or number of new referrals, you reward them with a gift of some kind. The gift can be a deep discount coupon, a free product or service, or something more expensive such as a trip. The purpose of this type of program is to get them excited about continuing to do business with you.

44. ACCEPT ONLY EXCELLENCE - If you expect average service performance, that is what you will get. Therefore, set your expectations of your employees high, both in the customer service area and all areas of your operation. Accept only excellent performance, and realize you must train your staff to achieve these levels of performance. Good enough should never be good enough.

45. EMPLOYEES ARE MEMBERS/CUSTOMERS, TOO - Never forget this. Employees are your internal members/customers, your first line of members/customers, and each of them has a customer somewhere in the value chain. Every employee must provide excellent customer service to every other employee so that they all can provide superior service to members/customers. This is the only way to guarantee customer satisfaction and retention. To put it simply, your employees will treat your customers the same way you treat your employees.

46. SHOW MEMBERS/CUSTOMERS YOU CARE - Send them thank you cards, holiday cards, and anything else you can to show them you care. Keep in constant contact with them so they never forget your name. Teach them that whenever they need something, they can come to you for it because you care. Spend time and money marketing your caring attitude to your members/customers. They will reward you with increased business.

47. MAKE SERVICE RESULTS VISIBLE - While it is true that what gets measured and rewarded gets done, it is also true that what is visible gets improved upon. Post your customer comment cards and letters for all members/customers and employees to see. Create a testimonial book of positive comments and letters for members/customers, prospects and employees to read. For employees, post their personal performance results in their lounge or locker room. Visibility enhances credibility, and

credibility is only enhanced by improved performance. Make service results visible so that your employees will constantly improve. Your members/customers will be the beneficiaries of this improved service.

48. GO THE EXTRA MILE OR TWO - When a customer wants something from you, give it to him or her. Then, do something extra. This little extra will go a long way to ensure their loyalty. For example, when you resolve a complaint to a customer's satisfaction, give them something extra to take away with them from the situation. Maybe it's a free class or a free personal training session. When you give them something of value that is extra and unexpected, they will be very grateful and you will now have a long term customer.

49. MARKETING AND CUSTOMER SERVICE GO HAND IN HAND - All of your marketing efforts should communicate your customer service message. In today's competitive marketplace, the only thing that differentiates fitness companies, clubs, facilities and programs from one another is the level and quality of their customer service. And, this is the major criteria people use to decide whether or not to continue doing business with a fitness company. Remember, that customer service is a very effective and powerful marketing tool, and that marketing is a very effective and powerful customer service tool. Combined, the two will help you keep your members/customers for life.

50. NOW, REVIEW EVERYTHING YOU HAVE DONE AND ARE DOING AND MAKE IT BETTER - Whatever you are doing now to service and satisfy your members/customers may not be sufficient to keep them tomorrow. A competitor will come up with a better product, program or class at a lower price that has more benefits and this will be offered with superior customer service. You have to stay ahead of your competitors. You must not only know what they are doing and going to do, you must also be proactive in your service efforts. Review everything you are doing to provide customer service then do whatever it takes to make it better. Remember that in the member/customer's mind, quality, service and continuous improvement often mean the same thing, or they are so tightly linked you cannot separate them. Meet or exceed this perception and the result will be a large base of loyal and long term members/customers.

These 50 tips to improving customer service in your fitness business should go a long way to help you become more profitable. You should also try to develop and implement additional service techniques that you can market so your business will continue to increase.

Success in the fitness industry is the result of a combination of effective marketing, which does not have to be expensive, and superior customer service. The final chapter gives you the means, methods and techniques to market your fitness programs and services at either no cost or a low cost.

Marketing Strategies and Tactics

Chapter 9

Strategies and Tactics For Marketing Success

Your marketing program is only as good as the promotional tactics and activities you use to implement it. Most small fitness centers, and even some larger ones, do not have the marketing and advertising budgets of some of the mega-chains. Therefore, the marketing, public relations and promotional implementation techniques presented in this section are all low cost or no cost to you. Don't let the cost fool you. One thing you can be sure of is that they all are effective.

The 130+ marketing techniques are presented in alphabetical order, like an index or catalog, to make it easier for you to locate a specific technique. The list is extensive, but it is not all inclusive. The goal here is to provide you with a variety of techniques you can use, as well as help you think of other techniques. In every case, you must adapt the recommendations and suggestions to the markets you serve, your current and prospective customers, and your resources to implement these techniques. Then, and only then, will you successfully market your fitness business.

Advertising

Before you embark on an advertising campaign for your fitness business, ask yourself: Is it really necessary to advertise? Then ask if you have enough money to have the campaign developed by professionals and can you sustain it for at least six months? If you answer no to either of these questions, then you should not advertise.

I am not a big fan of advertising programs for most small fitness centers anyway. That is because most fitness directors or centers create their own ads, do not track their effectiveness, do not target their markets correctly or effectively, and neglect to calculate their return on advertising investment. There are other marketing techniques you can use to achieve the same, or even greater results than with paid advertising. However, if you plan to advertise, follow these basic rules, regardless of whether the ad is for a newspaper, magazine, radio or television.

Have your headline copy scream a benefit at the reader, listener or viewer. If there is a subheading, have it reinforce the heading. Your copy should then support the headlines. Your copy should sell benefits, benefits, benefits, from the customer's perspective. Also, give them a problem and tell them how you are going to solve it for them. Don't worry about long or short copy. If you tell your story in an interesting manner, people will read it, listen to it or continue to watch it.

Make sure you have a response mechanism or a call to action in the ad. This invites or commands people to respond to your offer, either in writing or by telephone. Also, code your ads with a number or a symbol or a special department to call. This allows you to track the ads so you can determine their effectiveness along with your return on investment.

If the ads are not providing you with the responses you need to be financially profitable, then the ad campaign must be revised or abandoned. The only way you can determine this is through coding and tracking. Never believe that once the ad is created and placed, your work is done. That is a mistake. All ads must be coded and tracked for their effectiveness.

Advertising Agency

Many fitness centers develop and place ads themselves because they cannot afford an advertising agency. This is a good way to save money, especially if the agencies refuse to work with you because their commission on your ad placements (15%) would not net them enough profit for their efforts. Don't be discouraged by this. You can create ads that are just as good as an agency's ads by doing the following.

Use freelance writers and artists. There are enough of them available to you to help you create great looking ads that also draw business. Contact them through your yellow pages, have them come in and present their previous works to you, and give them a try. You may be pleasantly surprised that the ads you will develop are as good or better than those created by an agency.

Also, you can form your own in-house agency. It just requires a slightly different name from your regular fitness business. Then, you are entitled to all agency discounts that the big companies receive, including the commission on placement.

You can save 15% on almost every placement you make, as long as the media you are using pays a commission. Furthermore, as an agency, printers, copywriters and artists may work with you at a reduced price so that they can continue to get your business.

If you are going to use an ad agency, just make sure they present you with a marketing plan before they develop their advertising campaign for your fitness business. Or, make certain they have read your plan first. In either case, the marketing must drive the advertising. You must insist that the advertising they create for you will increase sales. It is never enough to just win advertising awards if sales and profits do not increase.

Remember, advertising is salesmanship in print, on the radio or television. Its one goal is to make you and your fitness business, not the agency, more successful. If the ads do not bring in more business, it is time to change agencies or to form your own.

Advertising Media

Advertising can be placed in print mediums, on radio or on television. Most small businesses use their local newspaper, with some radio. Check your rates for each. You may even be able to use cable television at certain times of the day, both for advertising and to have your own television show. Just make sure that if you are going to advertise or buy media time, the rates are what you can afford.

Print ads are usually of two types: classified or display. Display ads are the larger ads you see throughout the newspaper. They are the ones that are cluttered all over each other and make it hard to distinguish one from the other. If you are going to place a display ad, be unique and different enough, creative and innovative enough, so that the ad will stand out from the crowd.

You may also want to place a classified ad for your fitness center, product or service in the Sunday paper. Almost everyone reads the classifieds, and an ad that is slightly larger than the other classifieds will definitely draw attention. It is still less expensive than a display ad, and it has the chance of being seen by more people. Your paper may even have a special rate for a classified display ad. Look into this, as it will help you stand out from your competition.

Advertorials

Advertorials are paid-for advertisements in a newspaper or magazine that resemble an editorial or story. You write what appears to be an article about your fitness business and the newspaper or magazine places a disclaimer at the top stating that the piece is an advertorial.

This is a very effective method of promoting your business, if you can afford to purchase the space. People read this material and often perceive it as an article. This gives you more credibility than a typical display ad. However, the advertorial often requires more space than other ads and can be more expensive. If you squeeze an advertorial into a small space, it looks crowded and becomes difficult to read.

Consider the trade-offs if you plan to use advertorials Are they cost effective for the response rate you will receive? Also, how much do they add to your credibility? Does the advertorial increase your image, presence and visibility in the community so that more people join your center, or is the piece merely an ego enhancer for you? Is your story interesting enough that people will read it and then buy your membership or fitness product?

Articles

Publishing articles is one of the best possible ways to market yourself and your fitness business. Where you publish the article is not that important. It can be a major newspaper, a small local paper, a magazine, a trade or a professional journal. The important thing is to get the article published.

This provides you with credibility and the public instantly perceives you as an expert in the fitness field. If a publisher thought enough of you to publish your article on health and fitness, then you must be someone the public should know because you are an expert in fitness.

You will also be able to reprint these articles for use in a media kit or to send out as support material to corporate customers and prospects.

Make certain you write about your fitness business, or a topic related to health and fitness. Have your name printed on the byline and try to get the publication to print a brief bio of you at the end of the article. Remember that you want to use these articles to establish credibility and to inform the public about the fitness product or service you offer. Also, try to get the article published where it will be read by the types of people you want to serve.

Awards

People love to do business with award winners. After all, if someone thought enough of you to give you an award for something, you must be a winner. Right? And you must be among the best in the fitness field, otherwise why would you have received an award?

Publicize your fitness and business awards in every way possible. Inform the press about your achievements and certifications. Place the diploma, plaque or trophy on display in a conspicuous spot. Make certain everyone who enters your center can see them. Your clients, members and prospects who come in will be impressed.

Balloons and Blimps

One way to draw attention to your fitness center is to fly a giant balloon over the location with a sales message on the balloon. Many businesses do this when they have a grand opening. You should even consider this at other times during the year, especially when you are having a membership drive. It is so conspicuous that people must notice your location.

Other businesses have even rented blimps to fly over the area with their messages. Some blimp companies will rent you advertising time or space. While this may be an intriguing and unique concept to promote your fitness business, consider the cost, how many people will see the blimp and your message, and of those that do see it, how many will actually stop at your center to join?

Barter (Trade-Outs)

This is a great way to market your fitness business and not enough fitness directors take advantage of it. Basically, you are trading out your services for the goods and services of another business that will help both of you achieve your goals.

Barter as a marketing technique is very effective. It may not put money in the cash register, but it certainly can offer you many advantages over spending your own money. Consider it, and use it wisely.

Billboards

Roadside billboards are probably the premier form of outdoor advertising. They create high visibility for your fitness center and deliver a quick message about who you are and what you do to drivers. However, the rental of these billboards is not cheap. Some cost well over a thousand dollars a month. The billboard companies will help you design the board at no additional charge. They will also provide you with information on how many cars ride by your facility each day, along with the basic demographics of the area. This information is intended to help you decide where to place your billboard.

If you use billboards, keep your message to seven words or less. People driving by at high speeds do not have time to read long messages. Also, make certain there is a telephone number or an address on the board. While people probably will not stop to write it down, at least they will have some idea how to reach you.

Some of the larger fitness centers, and many companies in other industries, use billboards to establish and increase their name recognition and community awareness. This is an expensive method in and of itself, and it becomes even more expensive if the billboards do not bring you members. Ask yourself, what is the return on investment in the billboard and is it generating enough sales to more than cover its costs?

Board of Directors

Establish a board of directors for your fitness business. This can be an active board or an inactive one. An active board meets regularly with you and provides input into all aspects of the fitness business. An inactive board is usually used for their names and credibility only. The idea is to have people on your board who can help you succeed. Do not put family and friends on the board if they cannot bring you customers, members or leads, and give you advice on how to run the business.

Many companies that have a board of directors do not use them to their fullest capacity. Yes, they may help you set policy. But, as a marketer, you should view them as a resource. What other companies are they already doing business with that you are not? When can they introduce you, so you can get these corporations as clients?

You should ask influential people to sit on your board, and you should require them to bring one or two leads to each board meeting. Make it known that you will do the same for them. Use your board of directors to help you run your business and to expand your business.

Brochures

Brochures are an important part of any business, and especially a health and fitness business. They convey your positive image and marketing/sales message and represent you when you are not personally available to your members or prospects. They are a sales piece and an image builder. They keep you in the mind of your members or prospects. Therefore, if you are going to produce a brochure, make certain it is done professionally.

Too many fitness directors try to save money on their brochures by writing the pieces themselves and having them quick printed. This serves no beneficial purpose, and even costs you money in the long run. People will not want to do business with any fitness company that promotes itself with a cheap or unprofessional looking or poorly written brochure. Another problem of developing your own brochure is that fitness directors, being technical rather than sales people, write a technical piece rather than a sales piece.

Let professionals help you develop your brochures. Hire a professional graphics artist and copy writer. These people can take your ideas and turn them into sales messages that get you members. You will be pleasantly surprised at the result.

Your brochure should offer a benefit in the headline or on the first panel. Then, the copy should support that benefit and add value to it. Remember, people will buy what they perceive as a benefit and a value. Your brochures must tell them how what you offer will help them solve a problem, such as losing weight, or feeling better, such as reducing stress in their lives.

There are many types and sizes of brochures, and they all vary in cost. Determine what you want from your marketing plan, the sales message you want to promote, ask professionals to bid on the job, and then work closely with them. Just don't get in their way. These creative people will help you develop a brochure that you will be happy with and that will lead to increased business. You will be even more successful if the outside professionals you work with have experience developing brochures for the health and fitness field.

Budgets

You need to have one! I cannot say it any simpler or more direct. Too many fitness businesses never establish a marketing budget. They fly by the seat of their pants, take a shotgun approach to their marketing, and keep pouring money down the drain without ever knowing how much they are spending, what their return is, and what they are getting for the money.

Develop a marketing budget as part of your marketing plan. Stick to it as much as possible. If you have budgeted incorrectly, make changes based on sales and marketing goals. Never change a budget arbitrarily.

Review your budget monthly, quarterly and annually. Keep your staff informed about the budget and how well you are sticking to it. The difference between what you budgeted and actually spent is called the variance. A positive variance means you spent less than you budgeted and a negative variance means you spent more. Let the budget guide the marketing expenditures.

Bulletin Boards

Bulletin boards are a very effective marketing tool and very often, they are free. Check your local supermarket, restaurants, or even other businesses. Many places have bulletin boards where you can place your business card, a tear-off flyer or a brochure. And, the more bulletin boards you put your message on, the more people will begin to see it and recognize the name of your fitness business. While you may not receive a great deal of business from placing a business card or a flyer on an already crowded public bulletin board, you should expect a few calls. This will more than make the effort of placing the cards worthwhile.

You may also want to consider placing your business card or message on an electronic bulletin board that people access by computer. This is also an inexpensive method of promoting the fitness business. Furthermore, you will probably get a higher quality prospect list from these calls just because of the demographics of people who own computers, modems and use electronic bulletin boards.

One other suggestion. You may want to start your own bulletin board, and allow other businesses to place their message on it. Some companies even have elaborate, professionally designed boards where they sell space. The space is not expensive, but it more than pays for the cost of the board. Plus, you end up getting a free placement because your costs are covered by your other "advertisers".

Bundling *(also known as Piggybacking)*

Bundling, or piggybacking, is a marketing technique where two or more fitness products or services are sold as a package for less than the price of either alone. It is also used in direct mail, when one company already plans to do a mailing, and another company places something in the envelope at a reduced cost. Another example of bundling is a two for one sale, or buy one, get one free, or buy one and receive another item at half price. While these are all sales promotion techniques, and many fitness centers use them to sell memberships, they are variations of bundling.

Business Cards

People do not pay enough attention to their business cards. Business cards are among the most effective forms of marketing and they are often the most abused. You give out more business cards than anything else to promote yourself and your center. You should make certain that your card conveys your message and the appropriate image. Unless you are just starting out and cannot afford higher quality and professionally designed cards, then spending $10.00 for 1000 cards will provide your customers with a certain type of image, which you probably do not want.

DO NOT skimp on quality where your business cards are concerned. Also, make certain all your pertinent information is on the cards. The fitness business name should be prominent. If you have a logo, put it on the card. Your name, title, business address and all telephone numbers, including fax and mobile, should be on the card. If people cannot reach you or find you, how will you do business with them? How will they join your facility or participate in your programs?

Give out your cards every chance you get. Believe that everyone who has one of your cards is a potential member or can refer a potential customer to you. If giving someone your card makes you feel uncomfortable, ask them for their card first. They will be glad to give it to you and then you can offer them your card.

Here is another important point about business cards. You multiply and increase your marketing effectiveness by having business cards for all of your staff members. Many companies do this, but they tend to skimp on these "secondary" cards, such as those for receptionists. Give the staff people, especially your other fitness professionals, the same quality cards you have. Spend the extra money on them. They will become your best sales people and give out more cards to more people than you could imagine or ever hope to give out alone.

Business Meals

Some marketing experts tell you never to conduct business over a meal because the meal is distracting. I disagree. People have to eat, and if they do not want to hold a meeting over a meal, they will tell you. You should invite clients and prospects to a business meal, and then order according to your image as a fitness professional. Regardless of what the other person orders, you eat according to the image you are trying to project. And, since you did the inviting, you pick up the check.

Include business meals in your marketing plan and in your marketing budget. Business meals help people to relax, and they feel more comfortable telling you about their business and needs. The meal also makes it easier for you to close the deal. While most of my business is referral based, I can honestly tell you that the relationship is finalized more over lunch than at any other type of meeting.

Catalogs

If you are selling a fitness product, then catalogs are an excellent way to market your product. However, they can be very expensive if you are going to produce the catalog yourself. On top of that, you must add mailing list acquisition costs and postage. A more effective and less expensive method of selling through catalogs is to have your fitness product included in someone else's catalog. You may have to pay them a small fee or a percentage of sales, but this will be less expensive for you in the long run. They have already tested their format and their lists. All you have to do is supply them with the pictures and fulfill the orders.

Charities

Involvement with charities is an excellent way to gain a great deal of free publicity, visibility, community recognition and credibility. Select a charity to work with and then volunteer your time or donate products or services. Provide blood pressure screenings, cholesterol screenings, or conduct an exercise class as a fundraiser. You can inform the media about your actions. You should also be prepared to meet many other business people who are doing the same thing you are now doing: networking by assisting in a worthy cause.

Communication

There is not much to say about communication except that you must keep in touch with your clients, members and prospects. Write to them, call them, or better yet, go visit them: at home, at work or on the exercise floor. Never stay in your office for lengthy periods of time. Make sure they see or hear from you on a regular basis. Also, let them know what is going on with the fitness business. This will help you maintain their loyalty.

Confirmation Calls

Confirmation calls are used to remind a member or prospect of an appointment or a special event. You want to make certain they come to your facility. Confirmation calls also make people feel very special because it provides them with value-added customer service, and it shows you cared enough to call them.

Contests

Contests are great ways to get people involved with your fitness center and its programs. Contests can be sweepstakes, give-aways, promotional activities or anything else that requires people to participate in order to win something. The prize can be a free personal training session, a trip, a membership in your club, a free health promotion seminar, or anything else you can think of. The purpose of the contest is to get people involved with your fitness center or programs and to keep them coming back for more.

The success of the contest depends on its organization. The things you must consider include when and how long the contest will run, how many people (approximately) will participate, what printed materials will be needed and their cost, how contest information will be communicated to the members and the public, the type, cost and amount of the prizes, and how you will choose the winner(s). The contest itself will generate good visibility and publicity for you, as will the selection of the winner. Since this is also a newsworthy event, you should publicize it heavily.

Co-Op Advertising

There are millions, perhaps billions of dollars available every year for co-op advertising from vendors and manufacturers, yet the money goes unspent. This is because either fitness directors do not know about its availability or they do not know how to go about getting the money.

Co-op advertising is when you and one or more of your vendors or suppliers agree to jointly pay for advertising. They may pay you up front, after a certain amount of time has elapsed, and sometimes they pay you only after you spend a certain total dollar amount and show proof by furnishing them with the ads. The reason they give you this money is so that their product name is made visible by you in your community in conjunction with your own advertising and marketing of your fitness center.

The best way to receive money for co-op advertising is to ask for it. That's it, just ask. Tell the vendor about your marketing and advertising campaign and how it will benefit them. Your responsibility is to see that the advertising gets placed and the supplier's name is in the printed ad or mentioned on the radio or television.

There are two other forms of co-op advertising. One is discretionary funds and the other is vendor support. Discretionary funding requires you to send your supplier a proposal of your forthcoming marketing and advertising efforts. The proposal must include the exposure the supplier will receive from funding your effort. The reason this is called discretionary fund advertising is because the supplier is paying for the entire campaign, over and above any other monies that were designated for their own marketing campaign or co-op advertising.

Vendor support programs have vendors contribute to a marketing campaign and they receive mention in your advertising throughout the campaign. Vendor support differs from the discretionary fund advertising in that the former is usually tied to one specific event, such as a grand opening or charity fundraiser, while the latter usually is spread out over a longer period of time.

Co-Op Referral Lists

This is an arrangement between your fitness center or business and a non-competing business to trade customer (member) lists with each other. The purpose is to generate more business for both of you without taking business from either of you. Co-op referral lists often result when you join a networking group or a leads club. Businesses use this method as a reciprocal lead generation technique to help each other succeed.

Copy Cat Marketing and Advertising

This method of marketing is just what it says. You copy the best efforts of your competitors, but you must make sure that nothing they have made public is proprietary. Basically, you should not re-invent the wheel if you know something works well.

Coupons

This is a very popular form of sales promotion, and one of the best ways to get people to try your fitness center, product or service. You can put coupons in a newspaper or magazine, on a flyer, as part of a brochure, in your own coupon book and have other businesses pay a fee to be in there with you, or simply mail them or hand them out themselves. The purpose of a coupon is to offer a trial discount so a new customer will do business with you.

Some of the types of discount coupons include two for one purchases, a certain amount of money off on a purchase, free offers, buy one get the second at half price, and receive a free product or heavily discounted one with multiple purchases. You must decide on how coupons will work best for you. For the most part, they do work.

Coupons are relatively inexpensive to print. Place an expiration date on the coupon to create a sense of urgency to come in to see you and a code of some type to track the effectiveness and success of the coupon marketing campaign. Coupons are also a very effective method of marketing through cross promotions.

Cross Promotions *(Joint Venture Marketing)*

Cross promoting your fitness business with another business simply requires both of you to agree to pass out information or coupons to your respective customers so that they will do business with your partner in the promotion. The three simplest methods of cross promotion involve exchanging coupons, flyers, and displaying each other's merchandise. Two other, slightly more complicated methods, involve refrigerator cards and value cards.

Refrigerator cards are so named because you want the customer to paste the card on their refrigerator. The basic refrigerator card cross promotion involves two businesses, your fitness center and someone else, who contribute to a flyer. One side has a description of your fitness business with a coupon offer at the bottom. The reverse side has the same information about your partner's business but the information and the coupons are in the opposite position. This is to prevent a customer from cutting out your coupon and inadvertently destroying your partner's coupon.

One way to ensure repeated use of this program is to make each coupon good for 10 visits, so the customer has to keep the coupon on the refrigerator. Have your employees hole punch the coupon on each visit. Then, after the tenth visit, give the member something special, such as a free class or personal training session or a cholesterol screening.

The value card is really an extension of the refrigerator card. This cross promotion involves 6, 8, 10 or 12 businesses at the same time. Each business contributes a certain amount of money to the program and places their coupon on an 8.5 x 11 card stock paper. You then give each business, for example, 10 of them, 500 or 1000 of these value cards. This gives you 1000 x 9 or 9000 chances, plus a thousand of your own, of having new customers come into your fitness center because the other businesses are passing out coupons with your name on them.

Another way to increase your exposure with the value card is to print on the back of each coupon, "Compliments of . . .", and list the 10 businesses. If you add it up, you will be getting 10 impressions (mentions) on the back of card. If you print 10,000 cards, that is 10,000 impressions on the back, plus another 10,000 on the front. Where else can you get 100,000 impressions for only a few hundred dollars or less of an investment?

Customer or Member of the Month (Or Year)

This is a simple way to recognize your members/customers for their patronage. You simply purchase a plaque and each month, put a member's name on it. You must determine the selection criteria, but it can and should be very simple. For example, the member of the month can be someone who refers the most new members to your center or someone who purchases the most items or greatest dollar value, or someone who visits your facility and makes the largest number of purchases in a given month. Whatever criteria you decide upon, you do not want this to be a complicated issue.

You may also decide to give the winner a trophy, or their own plaque, or some other form of acknowledgment that they can take and keep. Doing this for your members will provide you with a loyal referral source who will continue to do business with you for a long period of time.

Customer Appreciation Programs

The customer of the month is one type of customer appreciation program. There are many others you can institute in your fitness business. A very simple one is a thank you card or note to new members or customers telling them you appreciate their business. Or, you can send the same thing to a customer who refers new business to you, thanking them for the referral. In fact, you should always do both.

Other types of appreciation programs include sending birthday and holiday cards to clients, members and customers. You can even send gifts to your extra special customers. This is done quite often around Christmas time, but you can also provide little, inexpensive gifts during the rest of the year to show them you care and appreciate their business. Another effort on your part that is appreciated by customers is when you call them to remind them of a training appointment, or you follow-up with them after they have called you regarding an inquiry or complaint. These confirmation calls go a long way toward establishing customer loyalty.

Customer Service

This could be the most important marketing tactic you can ever use. You must strive to satisfy your members and customers all the time. This means learning about and understanding their needs, wants and expectations, and then doing whatever it takes to meet those needs and wants and exceed those expectations. You should always go the extra mile and do the unexpected for your members or customers. This is especially true if you are trying to resolve a complaint. Remember that customers are the lifeblood of your business and the reason you are in business. You must do everything in your power to satisfy them. If you do not do this, your competitors will.

Customer Surveys

Surveys are an easy way to find out what your members/customers think about your fitness business, its products and services. These surveys do not have to be expensive. Some survey techniques include mailing written questionnaires to your members and hoping they will respond and return them, telephoning them and asking them a series of questions, and giving them a card to fill out while they are in the center or to mail back in.

An even simpler technique is to question them directly during or after their workout, or at the time they complete their purchase, or if they leave you without making a purchase. What did they like or dislike? What else would they like to see you do for them? Were they satisfied? These are just some of the questions you should ask. Also, you should use these surveys to solicit complaints from your customers. Then, use the complaints as opportunities to improve your business.

Demonstrations

Demonstrations are an excellent way to introduce people to your fitness product or service. You can provide free demonstration at malls, civic group meetings, residential facilities, and almost anywhere else you can think of. If you have a fitness-related product and provide free samples to get people to try it, that is the same as a demonstration. Sometimes, a free demonstration is the best and most effective way to get new customers. That is what one client of mine did with their exercise tubing, and now SPRI Products, Inc. is the world leader in rubber resistance exercise and rehabilitation devices.

Direct Mail

This is an area of fitness marketing that always receives a great deal of attention. The premise of direct mail is to make an offer to someone through the mail so that they will purchase what you are selling, such as a club membership or a series of health promotion classes. There have been some very successful direct mail campaigns that just used a letter from the marketer to the buyer, some that have been very elaborate and expensive while others were just very simple and inexpensive. Whatever type of direct mail program you plan to use, make certain it contains these basic components.

The mailing must contain at least a letter from you to the prospect, and preferably a brochure or catalog as a backup piece. You must then make the proper offer in your mail piece, meaning that you must motivate the reader to buy what you are offering. You can improve your success ratio with a current and accurate mailing list, which you can purchase from a list broker.

Some other suggestions include hand-writing the envelope instead of using mailing labels, sending the material first class with many smaller-valued stamps on the envelope to create the perception that you took a great deal of time to put the mailing together, and creating some sort of involvement with the piece.

This can be a scratch-off card, a tear-off coupon, or simply filling out a survey or calling a telephone number for a prize. You can also use a handwritten lift letter, which is a smaller piece of paper with a note, usually written by someone else, that tells the reader why they should buy, especially if they are considering not making a purchase or joining your facility. Quite often, lift letters help close the sale.

Remember that the most important thing in the direct mail piece is the letter, and it must state the nature of your business and make an offer. There have been many successful direct mail programs that only included a letter, but none or very few have ever been successful without a letter.

Direct Marketing

Direct marketing is a form of marketing that utilizes direct contact with the purchaser. This contact can be through direct mail, telemarketing and even personal sales. Direct marketing also requires the purchaser to become actively involved in the sales process in order to make a purchase and to become a more loyal customer or member. For example, if you operate a center and sell memberships, every person who comes in for a tour or membership information is exposed to your direct marketing efforts. The sales presentation is one way you promote your direct marketing, and your follow-up letters are another.

Direct Response Advertisements

ALL ADVERTISING MUST BE DIRECT RESPONSE! This means that customers fill out a coupon or a card and mail it in, or call you to order something, receive information or win a prize. You can even require the purchaser to visit your facility to claim their prize. Many clubs do this when they offer trial memberships, which consumers can receive only after they take a tour. The time-share real estate market uses something very similar in that you are informed you won a prize and can only collect it if you view their sales presentation. You, as the fitness marketer, are causing the prospect to make a direct response to your advertising.

Just remember to code each direct response ad with a name or a number so you can track its effectiveness. You do not want to keep spending money on direct response ads that do not make sales for you.

Directories

Directories are a good way to list your fitness business and your name for people to see. Directories can be regional, national or local, part of a civic organization or professional group, and they can also be used as a marketing vehicle if you choose to advertise in them. When people see your name listed over and over again in a directory, it creates a feeling of security on their part because you are perceived as credible and in business for a long time. If you were not credible, would the directory allow you to be listed? Choose your directories carefully, as they sometimes cost money and they are all not for everyone.

Displays

Displays are used a great deal in stores by suppliers to promote their merchandise. They are also used by manufacturers and vendors at trade shows. You should set up various displays in your fitness center to promote programs, classes, and special events. The purpose of a display is to attract people's attention and to get them to buy what is being displayed.

There are very elaborate displays and there are some very inexpensive ones. Displays can be simple signs, table tops, bulletin boards, and free standing, as you see at major trade shows. The display should be eye catching and informative at the same time. Also, you can use a display to enhance a sales presentation. You must decide on the type of display you want to use in the center and then make it work for you.

Distribution Channels

These are the ways in which you make the public aware of your center, products or services so that they can buy from you. Develop new, creative, unique, innovative and improved distribution channels for whatever you are selling, especially since everyone uses the standard methods. How will you be different? Coming up with a new distribution channel might possibly turn your fitness business into an overnight success.

Door Hangers

These are the plastic bags or hooked pieces that people place on your front door knob. While you may not like a door hanger on your front door when you come home, you must admit they attract your attention. They are also fairly inexpensive, as they usually include a flyer that makes a special offer from one or a number of businesses.

You can set up your own door hanger program and have others pay to participate. Just figure out your costs, get other businesses to sign up, and use those monies to pay the people who distribute the door hangers. You may want to use high school students as your representatives. If you participate in someone else's door hanger program, make certain they can guarantee you a specific number of pieces get placed. If they can't, do not get involved as you will be wasting your money.

Expanded Business Hours

This may seem intuitively logical, but many companies never work beyond the traditional 8:00 - 5:00 or 5:30. You should make your fitness business convenient and accessible to customers. Quite often, people will do business with someone just because they are open earlier or later. Banks learned this a long time ago and now stay open later on Fridays, which is a traditional pay day. Clubs open at 5:00 or 6:00 a.m. and stay open until 9:00 or 10:00 at night, and some are even open 24 hours. Find out if your customers want you to expand your hours of operation, then calculate your costs against your potential revenues.

Fact Sheet

A fact sheet is a one page description of your fitness business, product or service. It can be a flyer with facts about your business, or it can be a more formal, printed piece. More often than not, a fact sheet is used to support a presentation or provide a customer with some additional information. Your fact sheet should list the features, advantages and benefits of working with you in addition to the basic descriptions mentioned above.

Fairs

Fairs come in all types and sizes. There are state, regional and local fairs. There are business fairs, health fairs, and expositions. There are also community display fairs. You must decide if you want to display your fitness business at one of these fairs. Your investment is one of time, a display, booth costs and printed material to give out. You may also want to provide free samples or demonstrations. Your activities at a fair are similar to your work at a trade show. You should also consider displaying at fairs that are not health and fitness related. This shows the public that you truly are a business, and you can attract members and participants from a market that was previously unavailable to you.

Flyers

Flyers are the least expensive way to inform the public about your fitness business. Flyers can be used to announce new classes, new programs, special product sales, special events, new products, discounts, to provide coupons, fundraisers, or just to create a visible presence for you in the community.

You can make up flyers on your computer or have them typeset and run off at a printer. The choice depends on what you are trying to accomplish, how much you want to spend, and the image you are trying to create. There are numerous businesses that have been successful with just handwritten flyers, but you would probably want yours to look more professional.

Flyers can be made more eye-catching if you use photos or graphics. People like to see pictures, since that is the way their minds work. Pictures that tell your story will have a greater effect on potential customers than just words. So, try to combine pictures with your descriptions to make your flyers more effective.

Free Anything

Giving something away **FREE**, such as a sample product or an initial consultation, is an excellent way to get someone to do business with you. Once they have tried your product or experienced your service, then it is up to you to get and keep them as a customer. Most people are glad to try something for free, but they are reluctant to pay for something new and untried. Therefore, consider giving it away to get more back later. As contrary as it may seem, the word "FREE" in an ad or marketing communication still draws more people than any other type of offer.

Gift Certificates

Gift certificates are often used to attract new members/customers, to get current customers to purchase more, or to have current members give the gift certificates to family and friends for special occasions. People like to receive gift certificates, especially around the holidays. You should make them available at that time, but they should also be available all year long. The concept is easy to implement, and I suggest these certificates be printed. You can leave the amount off and just write it in, or, if you have a big gift certificate program, print them up with different amounts. Then, you just have to fill in the person's name.

Grand Opening

This is very effective if you are a new fitness business. Wait about two to three months after you have opened, work all the bugs out, and then plan your grand opening. Make it interesting, festive and fun. Invite current members and prospective customers. Inform the media about your event to get additional publicity. Give away products, prizes, coupons, gift certificates, memberships, equipment and anything else you can think of to get people to try your facility, product or service now and in the future.

You can also turn the grand opening into an annual event. In subsequent years, you can host an open house. Do everything the same way. The goal is to attract new business while keeping your current customers loyal.

Grand Prize Drawing

This is one of the best ways to develop a mailing list. Either purchase a prize yourself to give away, or work with another business, say a travel agency, to offer their prize to your customers. Set up registration boxes in various locations, including in your center. Have a final entry date, draw the winner, contact the winner, announce it to the media, and try to get coverage for the day you award the prize in person. Grand prize drawings, or contests of any kind, tend to attract people to your fitness business, many of whom you can convert to customers and members.

Guarantees

Guarantees will help you differentiate your fitness business from your competitors. Whatever type of guarantee you offer, lifetime, money back, or exchange during a certain time period, just make certain that you honor that guarantee. While guarantees can be very attractive to buyers, they can also turn customers away if they are not honored.

Your type and length of guarantee tells customers the confidence you have in your business. There will be times when you have to honor many guarantees simultaneously, but the goodwill this will generate will be more than worth the investment. Consider your business, what it does for the customer, and then decide on the guarantee you will provide. Just make sure you can honor it.

Help Lines or Hot Lines

Many businesses have instituted 800 and 900 telephone help or hot lines for their customers. This is very effective and not that expensive, especially if you deal on a regional or national basis. You can even establish a local help or hot line that gives out health and fitness information.

Train your personnel to answer the questions that customers may have about your fitness business in a courteous and friendly manner. Teach your customers that they can call the help line any time for assistance. It is even better to offer this assistance, whether it is informational or technical, such as with computers, for free. You will have more people using the line, but they will also start to refer more people to your fitness business because of this service. In this way, the cost of the help line more than pays for itself from the increased membership and product sales.

Your help line can also be pre-recorded messages about health and fitness topics. Callers access a particular topic by pressing a code on their telephone, then they hear a recorded message. Make certain that you promote your fitness both at the beginning and end of the message.

Host or Hostess

Having a host or hostess at your fitness center is an excellent way to make members feel comfortable when they enter the facility. This person is not a receptionist, but actually someone who meets and greets people as they enter the club. This person's role is the same as that of a party host; to make the people feel at home.

You can either hire a host or hostess, as they often do in restaurants, or you can have a volunteer fill the role. Some of the best hosts and hostesses have been retired men and women who like to be with people and want to fill up their time. Having one of these experienced people working for you will give you a warm, friendly and inviting atmosphere to your fitness center. And, just to show your appreciation, if these people are volunteers, allow them to use the facilities for free.

In-Service Training (see Staff Training, also)

Employee training is probably the most overlooked and under utilized marketing technique. Training programs are relatively inexpensive when compared to the returns. Training employees to do their jobs better, or cross training them to help out in other areas of the club, makes employees feel that they are more valuable to the company. They will produce more, and market your company to more customers. Remember that your two best sales staffs include satisfied customers and happy employees.

Inserts

Inserts, and free standing inserts, are used to attract attention to a special offer by a fitness center or service provider. They are either attached to some other advertising piece or they are unattached within another piece. Businesses use inserts because they are usually less expensive than traditional advertising. Inserts are often similar to flyers and can also be used as such and contain coupon offers.

Inserts are most often used with print media, such as newspapers, magazines, catalogs, newsletters, and almost anything else that a customer would read. This form of marketing can be very effective if it works, or it can be very costly if it does not generate the business.

Internal Marketing

You must market to your employees first, before you do anything else. Then, you must market to your current customers. These are your two greatest sources of new and repeat business. Treat these internal markets properly and then communicate your message to the outside public.

Image

Image advertising can be very expensive. Many new fitness companies decide to embark on an image building advertising campaign, only to abandon it because of its cost. Although every fitness business needs a public image, the smart companies build their images through the creation of marketing awareness, recognition, credibility, reliability and longevity. A variety of techniques are used, but wise fitness businesses do not rely heavily on image advertising. They tend to use more public relations, networking and community visibility than anything else.

Incentives

Incentives have proven very successful in motivating salespeople to achieve greater sales volumes, and these same incentives can also motivate your staff to perform better, increase productivity, and serve as your best marketing representatives. Incentives do not always have to be monetary, but some money rewards usually help. Incentives can be gifts, trips, dinners, paying for attendance at regional or national conventions, or anything that is out of the ordinary reward structure for your fitness business. Just develop a program that ties the incentives to performance and reward accordingly.

Interns

Interns are a very reliable source of quality employees. College students in health and fitness fields must complete an internship in order to graduate. Contact your local college and work with them to develop an internship program with your fitness center. Most undergraduate internships are not paid, while graduate interns often receive some compensation. The details can be worked out with the school. The important thing is to bring interns into your fitness business, train and treat them as you would any regular employee, and make them part of your marketing effort.

Joint Venture Marketing

In many cases, joint venture marketing is similar to cross promoting between two or more businesses. With joint venture marketing, you work with a non-competing business to jointly market your products or services. You share in the costs of the marketing efforts. The revenues generated from this program can also be shared, but more often than not, they go to each business separately.

The purpose of joint venture marketing programs is to attract customers to your fitness business from a source you were previously unable to reach, and to provide customers for your joint venture partner. This reciprocal marketing relationship breeds confidence and trust among the businesses and their respective customers. The best way to start a joint venture marketing program is to ask a neighboring business if they would like to participate. You can then use flyers, discount coupons or books, and value cards as some possible ways to make this program work.

Lead Boxes

The health club industry is light years ahead of other industries in using lead boxes to generate mailing lists and traffic flow. Everywhere you go, you see these lead boxes that invite you to register to win a free two week membership, or some other prize. Combining lead boxes with give-aways is a great way to get people to notice your fitness business and to show their interest. The most important thing about a lead box program is the follow-up. Make sure that when you collect these lead boxes full of names and telephone numbers, you call these people and try to get them to come into your center or participate in your programs. If you do not follow up, you have wasted your time with this type of program.

Leads Clubs

Some entrepreneurs have established leads clubs, where non-competing business owners and sales people meet on a regular basis to exchange leads with each other. Find out if there is such a club in your area and join it. Leads clubs typically allow only one person per industry to be a member, so there are no conflicts. Since most fitness professionals I know do not circulate outside the industry that often, this may be an excellent marketing tool for you. The club provides you with a rich source of prospects whom you would otherwise never have known about. Again, the important thing is to follow up on these leads.

Letters of News

Everyone is familiar with newsletters. Your club probably sends one to its members. In fact, people get so many newsletters, they hardly ever have the time to read them all. Make your newsletter stand out by sending it as a letter of news.

This is a personalized letter to your member/customer that contains the same information that would appear in a traditional newsletter. The only difference is this information is written in letter form and signed by you as the fitness director. People are more likely to read a "personal" letter than an impersonal newsletter. (Newsletters obviously serve a valuable purpose in the business marketing world. Just look at the number of newsletters that are published, plus the prices people are willing to pay to receive this information.)

Letters to the Editor

These appear each day in your newspaper. Have you ever considered the publicity value to your fitness business of you writing a letter to the editor? You sign it with your name and your company name. Just don't make the letter seem like a blatant advertisement for your fitness business. Follow up on a health related issue or something the newspaper reported on earlier in the fitness field. Give your opinion, or state the position your company has on the issue. Write enough of these and it begins to look like you have your own column. The result will be increased credibility and visibility. Also, when your letters are published, cut them out and place them in your publicity kit.

Leveraging

This is a simple marketing tool whereby you ask your current members and suppliers to introduce you to new business, or provide you with referrals. Leveraging works especially well with suppliers and vendors since they do not want to lose your business. You may not realize it, but you leverage yourself every time you ask someone if they know of someone else who can benefit from the fitness services you offer. Since you do it to friends, families and customers, why not ask your suppliers for the same type of information? You might be surprised at how many of them are willing to help you.

Logo

Every fitness business should have a logo. The logo identifies you to the public and provides a direct or hidden message about your fitness business.

Make sure the logo says what you want it to say. If your goal is for the logo just to make an impression so people will remember your company name, then create one that will achieve that goal for you. Pay a graphics artist, if necessary, to make your concepts come to life.

The logo for my company is facing "G's". It appears in the background on business cards and stationary. This, then, makes someone look twice. The first time they look at our printed material, they realize something was there but they are not quite sure. Now, they have to look again, and this gives another chance to imprint the

GERSON GOODSON, Inc.

Marketing Management Training

Richard F. Gerson, Ph.D.
President

P.O. Box 1534 Safety Harbor, Florida 34695
Tel/Fax 813-726-7619 Pager 813-449-4611

company logo and name in their memory. The logo also provides a subliminal message about how we do business: face to face in a mutually beneficial relationship.

Mailing Lists

Mailing lists are an effective direct marketing tool and they are easy to obtain. There are many list houses that produce a mailing list for you according to your specifications. Of course, there is a cost associated with this service. The advantage is that it lets you target your marketing efforts in a very precise manner.

You can also develop you own in-house mailing list from your members, customers and shoppers. Then, you can send them periodic information on your fitness programs and services. Whether you work with purchased lists or in-house lists, they must be accurate and up to date. If you use quality lists, you will have a very effective, and fairly inexpensive marketing tool.

Marketing Plan

You must have a marketing plan in order to succeed. In fact, you must have a written marketing plan, and this can be one of three types. The first is the formal and comprehensive marketing plan that spans about 50-75 pages. The next is an informal plan that just gives enough information and direction on where you are going and how you are promoting your fitness business. The last type is merely a listing of tactical action plans, usually for a 90-day period. Whatever you do, make certain you have at least one of these three written down.

Market Research

Most fitness businesses do not conduct market research because they think they cannot afford it or they believe they do not know how to do the research properly. They are wrong on both counts. There are many free sources of information about the fitness industry, your competitors and your customers. You just have to know whom to ask for it and where to find it.

The first place you start is with the library. They can help you gather information in a very effective and comprehensive manner on almost anything you need related to the fitness industry. And, this service is free. More often than not, this information is similar to the information a market research firm would provide at a cost of thousands of dollars. Another free market research technique is to ask your customers and employees about your fitness business. Also, have courage and ask your competitors about your business and theirs. Listen to their suggestions, and make the appropriate improvements.

There are two types of market research: primary, which you collect by yourself for a specific project and which can become very expensive; and secondary, which is information collected for another purpose but that can be used by you at any time. This information is collected through personal interviews, telemarketing, surveys, and intercepts, where people are stopped in a club, mall or parking lot and asked to answer a few questions.

Marketing research can only be valuable to your fitness business if the information you collect is acted upon. You do not want to have volumes of data and do nothing with it. You must do something with the information you have collected. Sometimes the results are not what you wanted or expected. However, this can be very valuable if it prevents you from entering a market or offering a fitness product or service that no one will buy.

Fitness companies use market research to test new products and services, to test membership prices, to test program acceptance, to determine customer satisfaction, and to find out how customers feel about their current products. Do your research, pay attention to the data and the results, and you will be glad you did.

Marriage Mailers

Marriage mailers are mailings that promote several businesses at one time. Usually, there is a central mailing house or distributor who puts the program together, sells the clients on the value of placing their coupon in this marriage mailer because it is highly targeted to a geographic service area (by zip code) and then prints up and mails all the pieces. The key is to make your individual piece stand out from everything else that is in the envelope. You do this by using colored paper, larger print, a different size flyer, making an outrageous offer, or anything else you can think of. Some marriage mailer companies you may be familiar with include Val-Pak, Advo, and Stuff-It.

Memberships and Networking

These two tactics are put together because they are often identical. You should join as many local, civic and professional associations as you can afford, both financially and time-wise, and that can benefit your fitness business. The contacts you will make through these memberships can provide tremendous support for your fitness business. Furthermore, your visibility and credibility are increased by your contact with people in different organizations and from different fields. Just make sure that your net is working.

Your networking sphere expands when you attend the association or organization meetings. Sponsoring some of the organization's events is also a great way to network and make new contacts. The recommendation here is not to be a passive member of something. Make your membership count. Make it work as a marketing tool that will generate new business for you and help your current members/customers.

Name

If you have nothing else to work with when marketing your fitness business, make certain your name conveys the proper marketing message. Customers should know who you are and what you do simply by seeing or hearing your name.

Many business owners like to have their own name as the company name, in whole or in part. This is very true with professional service providers. You must then consider a longer company name to convey the message, or you can use a subtitle, as we do: Gerson Goodson, Inc.: Marketing, Management and Training Services. Now, everyone we meet knows who we are and what we do.

Networking

As mentioned previously, one of the ways you network is to join clubs and organizations. The basic premise of networking is to establish and increase your sphere of influence and visibility within the community. You should meet and greet as many people as possible. It is almost like running for political office where you must shake hands, pat backs and kiss babies. The more of this you do, the greater your chances of receiving new members or customers through referrals.

Remember, the person with whom you network today may not become your customer, but he or she may refer someone to you, or refer you to someone who refers someone to you. You never know how far your network will extend. Therefore, treat everyone you meet as a potential referral source from your network. Also, treat them as a possible customer.

New Business Requests

There are many fitness companies that do not grow or succeed simply because the owners or directors never asked for new business. This is a very simple procedure where you ask your current customers to recommend someone they know who can benefit from your product or services. Your request can be in person or in writing. It is just another way of requesting referrals.

There is a way to make this more effective and that is to describe a potential customer or an ideal customer to your referral source. Sometimes, people who are asked to refer someone just can't think of anyone off the top of their head. However, if you describe the characteristics of your desired customer, these people become quite capable of thinking of someone. All you have to do is ask.

New or Short-Term Services

This is a marketing tactic where you diversify your offering for a brief period of time, perhaps by providing a special membership or program sale. You may offer free introductory health promotion classes to get people into your facility in order to sell them a membership. Or, you may provide these classes free with every membership that is purchased. The purpose of a short-term service offering is to generate revenues quickly.

Newsletter

Newsletters are an excellent way to keep in touch with your clients and prospects. The letter of news mentioned earlier is just one form of a newsletter, and you must decide on your most effective method of communication.

Newsletters provide information in a short, concise fashion. They help readers acquire knowledge that they probably otherwise would never receive because they do not have time to read the original sources. Fitness businesses that send newsletters do this to keep in touch with their clients, maintain visibility and provide a value-added service.

Newsletters can be very elaborate or very simple. If you are just starting a company newsletter, either to clients, prospects, employees, or employees, or everyone, keep it simple. Both sides of an 8.5" x 11" page is sufficient to begin with. Lay out your information so it is easy to read and follow. Use a big headline followed by two or three columns. Use only two or three print sizes in the body of the newsletter. Actually, all your copy should be one print size and the section headings and subheadings should be another.

Newsletters are a great way to stay in touch and to remind clients who you are. There is obviously an expense associated with producing a newsletter, especially if you are providing it for free. However, the expense is just a cost of doing business and the return on this investment can be significant.

If you plan to start a newsletter but do not know how, seek help from a professional. Check with a graphics artist, a printer, a communications specialist, a public relations or marketing consultant. Also, when you send the newsletter, have it do double duty by including your own sales insert on a separate piece of paper in the newsletter. You will be pleasantly surprised at the increase in membership or product sales you receive from this newsletter insert.

Novelty Items

Novelty items are unique "toys" that people would never really buy for themselves, but that they really would like to have. You provide these novelty items to them as an adjunct to your fitness product or service. The item enhances your primary product or service and is basically a memory reinforcer so that they will remember you when it comes time to purchase again. Some types of novelty items include pens, key chains, calendars, address books, coasters, paper weights, watches and clocks.

Off Pricing

This marketing technique is used most often when business is slow. Fitness centers advertise an off-price membership sale to the public to try to generate revenues. A more effective and less expensive off-price approach would be to send a letter to your current and former members/customers informing them of a special sale just for them. All products (memberships, services, classes, etc.) will be reduced in price (off-price) for a short period of time as a way of thanking them for their business. You can even go further in the letter by stating that this off-price sale will not be advertised to the public. You will not only generate sales, but you will also generate a great deal of good will and loyalty from your members/customers.

One Minute Messages

This works very well for fitness professionals because they always have so much information to give to clients. The premise is to spend an extra minute with each member/customer telling them about something that is of interest. It can be a message on health, an upcoming sale, or a new product that will be coming out. The point is to personally invest one extra minute to market yourself and your fitness business, and have your employees do the same.

Packaging

Your packaging can make or break you, especially in the fitness industry. Often times, your packaging is you, your staff and your facility. If each and all of these do not present the "packaged" image the public expects from the fitness industry, you will go broke.

Many years ago, I had a professional colleague who was the health promotion director for a government agency. This person had trouble getting employees to attend classes on stress management, weight control and smoking cessation. She asked for my marketing advice and the first thing I did was asked the employees what prevented them from attending. They told me it was the appearance of the HP director. This person was highly anxious, overweight and smoked. With packaging like this, it is no wonder the employees did not attend classes.

With fitness programs and services, the packaging is the image you, as the service provider, present. Remember that as you go on your next prospect call or client visit. You are both the packaging and the service rolled into one. Package yourself and your employees well, and you should see an increase in revenues.

Personal Sales

Personal sales is the one form of marketing that you can control totally, and that contributes directly to your success in the fitness business. Everyone sells all the time, yet many people are afraid to sell or believe that they do not sell. This is especially true of technical and clinical people such as fitness professionals. Yet, you and your employees must realize that without a sale, there is no business.

The first step in being successful at personal sales is to believe in yourself and what you are selling. With health and fitness, that should be very easy. We have all been accused, at one time or another, of being fanatical and evangelical about the lifestyle. Channel this into enthusiasm for what you are selling. Then, you just have to be yourself with the client.

There are volumes of material on how to be a successful salesperson. Follow these simple steps and you will be able to condense all that information. First, know yourself and your fitness product. Dress professionally. Establish rapport and confidence with your prospect. Try to learn and understand what the prospect needs, wants and expects. Ask open ended questions and let them answer. Listen more than you speak. Communicate that you want to establish a relationship, not just a one time sale. When you listen, and communicate your desire to help them in an honest and sincere way, people will sell themselves.

Per Inquiry or Per Order Advertising

Many fitness companies simply cannot afford the high costs of advertising. Per inquiry or per order advertising is a way to reduce those costs. Work with the advertising medium or supplier and provide them with a specific amount of money or a percentage based on each inquiry or membership sale that you get as a result of your ads with them. You are essentially paying them from money you hope to earn with a per inquiry approach, and from money you are definitely earning with a per order approach. These two approaches work very well with direct marketing of a fitness product, program or service.

Advertisers may be reluctant not to get their money up front. However, you must show them that they have the potential to make more money with one of these approaches. When you do this, you may be able to advertise in places and ways you could never have afforded otherwise. Everyone involved in these types of marketing techniques must be able to "see the future", because that is where the payoff is.

Phone Hold Messages

Many fitness businesses have to place their customers on hold on the telephone for various periods of time. These fitness businesses also tend to play radio music during that time. What happens if the radio is playing an ad for your competitor? Then, you are basically paying for your customer or prospect to listen to your competitor's ads.

Phone hold messages play your advertising and marketing messages to customers while they wait on hold. They only hear about your fitness business, your programs, classes and services, and nothing else. There are companies that just set up phone hold message systems, or you can call your local telephone company. If you are not going to take advantage of phone hold messages, then don't play anything at all.

Piggybacking

Piggybacking is a simple marketing technique where you get involved with an already successful event or promotion. Many fitness businesses, and other industries also, use piggybacking when they work with a charity that has an annual fundraiser. The fundraiser is an established, successful event, and now the fitness business has chosen to become a part of it. The cost is usually minimal, the visibility is high, and the credibility is instant.

Piggybacking can also be used in other ways and with other businesses. You would usually want to piggyback with non-competing businesses, but sometimes it is beneficial to work with your competitors on a program. Take a look around your community and see if there are any events, programs or promotions that you can become part of. Even though you will be doing the piggybacking, you still must contribute your time, effort and some money to the success of the program.

Pooling

This is where a group of businesses, both in and out of the fitness industry, pool their resources and funds to promote themselves to attract new customers. Basically, each business is spreading out the cost of marketing to the public. You can pool marketing efforts with both competitors and non-competitors. The key is to increase your buying power, if you are advertising, and to increase your visibility and penetration in the marketplace by pooling your resources. Another way to describe pooling is that several businesses are cooperating to increase their chances of success.

Positioning

This is not so much a marketing implementation technique as it is part of the marketing plan and the foundation for all your implementation techniques. Positioning is the place you hold in the minds of your customers in comparison to your competitors. Are you the fitness market leader or follower in your area? Do you offer quality service and programs or poor service and programs? Are your membership prices the highest or the lowest, or in the middle? These are some of the ways to position your fitness business. Keep in mind that positioning your business properly and then targeting your efforts to support that position will ensure your success.

Preemptive Marketing

Here is a technique that carries a great deal of weight with the public but is used very sparingly by businesses in any industry. Preemptive marketing means you are either the first to do something, or at least, the first one to announce you have done something. For example, let's assume that every one of your competitors is offering personal training for a similar price. While they all advertise this service, none of them are telling the public why PT may be better for their fitness levels. You decide to tell the whole story, including benefits such as more personalized attention, faster fitness results, increased knowledge, and whatever else you can think of. People will perceive you as the best facility to go to for PT because you told them the whole truth about personal training in a way they can understand.

People like to do business with winners, others who are first. Just let them know that you are the first in the fitness field to do something, and they will want to work with you. Of course, you must be able to support your claim that you are the first.

Premiums

Premiums are inexpensive, high perceived value add-ons to a regular purchase, or they are free gifts to a client or prospect or an employee. Premiums connote extra value, and they are provided as an incentive to continue to do business with your fitness company. In fact, premiums are quite often referred to as premium incentives.

You may already be offering premiums such as club tee shirts, shorts, pens or other specialty advertising items that promote your club and make your members/customers feel special. If so, you should continue. If you are not offering premiums, you should consider using them.

Press Kit (Media Kit)

This is essential for any fitness business to have. It does not have to be very expensive, but it must be professional.

Your press kit contains information about your fitness company, its key employees, the products or services you offer, your own or the company's achievements, and other information that is pertinent or interesting to the media. This can be reprints of articles you have written or that have been written about you or the fitness center or business. The press kit can also contain testimonial letters from satisfied customers, along with a picture of the person, product or service you are trying to promote.

The press kit is used whenever you need to send out more information than is covered in a press release, or when the media requests more information from you. It is an extension of your corporate image. That is why you must make certain the kit looks very professional. If you cannot develop one yourself, seek the assistance of a marketing or public relations professional.

Press Release

For the cost of a stamp, you can inform all the media in your area, and even nationally, about a newsworthy event concerning your fitness business. This can be a new hire, a promotion, a special event, an award, or anything else the media may want to publicize for you for free.

Press releases should be short, one or two pages, and should provide the reader with enough information to arouse their interest. You want the press release to motivate the reporter to contact you for more information and to do a story on you. The best way to do this is to put your newsworthy information into a format that the press is already comfortable with.

Your press release begins with a heading that identifies it as a press, media or news release. You should have a publication date, contact person and day and evening contact telephone numbers on the top of the release. Then, you should specify when the release can be used, either with a date or by saying "For Immediate Release". The sample press release on page 38 shows the layout and format for a well-written piece.

Your headline should be short and capture attention. You then start to tell your story with the most pertinent and important information first. You must basically answer the questions who, what, when, where, how and why in this release. You adapt the order of presenting this information to fit the lead and the type of media you are sending it to, as well as to make certain you include all the pertinent information.

As you write the release, you go from the specific to the more general, or from the most important to the least important. When editors use your release, they will use it on a space available basis. This means they will cut out any information they do not perceive as valuable. If you write the release in this standard format, they will cut from the bottom up.

One way to view the format is as an inverted pyramid that is wide at the top and narrows as you approach the bottom. That is how your press release will be read and edited.

Here are some other suggestions regarding press releases. Use them wisely and judiciously. Send them only when you have something newsworthy to publicize, otherwise, editors will get tired of seeing your company name and stop using your information. Try to schedule newsworthy events on a regular basis so you can send press releases every other month. Then, follow up with a telephone call to the editor to find out if they received the release, if they have any questions, and if they plan to use the release. Be courteous. Do not make a pest of yourself, either with the releases or the telephone calls. The editors appreciate your sending them the information, but they can only use it on a space available basis. If it is very newsworthy, you can be sure they will make the space available.

Top 10 Health Fitness Topics for Press Releases

Here is a list of the top 10 topics in the health and fitness fields that interest editors when you send a press release. Of course, you should adapt this list as you get to know your media contacts personally and find out exactly what interests them.

1. Tie-ins with the health, fitness or medical news of the day.

2. Staging a special event, such as a grand opening, open house, or hosting an author or fitness celebrity.

3. Providing the community with useful information. This should be very easy for any fitness director to do.

4. Forming a committee to solve a problem in the community, such as no health promotion classes for school children.

5. Giving away an award or scholarship to a staff member or a community resident.

6. Making a prediction about something related to people's health.

7. Celebrating an anniversary.

8. Doing something incredible or very special, for yourself, for or with others, and especially for the community or a non-profit charity.

9. Giving away food, especially around Thanksgiving and Christmas.

10. Any type of success story, especially overcoming hardship, such as a physically challenged person who rehabilitates himself or herself at your facility.

Can you think of other topics that would be of interest.
Fill them in in the spaces below.

11.

12.

13.

14.

15.

Price Competitively

Competitively pricing your memberships, programs, product or service is a marketing tactic that is often overlooked. The goal here is not to be the low cost leader, but to provide perceived value at a competitive price. Quite often, a fitness business just selects a price for their offering without considering the marketplace or the market value. These facilities are usually the first to go out of business.

You must price your products or services to be competitive and to provide a value to the customers. You should then give added service at no charge, such as more personalized attention, expanded hours of operation, or free classes. Your customers will perceive your fitness center and business as not only providing a good value, but as someone they want to do business with on a continuing basis.

Sometimes, you just have to price things low and make up the difference on volume. Of course, if you are the only fitness business in the marketplace, then you could probably charge reasonably high prices and the members/customers will pay it. Once other businesses join you, you must become competitive.

Public Service Announcements (PSAs)

Every radio and television station provides the community with public service announcements. These are free announcements on the air informing the public of a free service you are providing. You may be offering to do some community service or charity work, such as leading an exercise class as a fundraiser, or you may be giving away fitness products or food. Informing the media of these free events and efforts on your part will lead to public service announcements. The resulting visibility and credibility only serve to enhance your fitness business. You should use PSAs as wisely and judiciously as you use your press releases.

Quality

This is more of a way to compete than a marketing tactic, but it is becoming more central to successful marketing than ever before. People are looking for value for their money, especially when they use discretionary funds to purchase fitness memberships and attend classes and workshops. They measure value in the quality of their purchase. Does it (you) do what you said it would do? You must promise quality, deliver quality, and then deliver more of it. This is the only way to compete on the quality dimension. Also, remember that quality is defined by the customer, not the provider.

Radio Programs

Check out your local AM talk show stations. They are often willing to sell time slots to you to air your own radio show. The cost is usually reasonable, and the returns can be extraordinary. Being host of your own radio show gives you instant credibility and the ability to reach a large, highly targeted audience. The key to making this work is that you have to know when and how you promote your own fitness business during the show. Of course, you also must have the funds available to purchase the time.

You should also contact the talk show hosts and try to become a guest on their shows. Health and fitness topics are always of interest to the general public, and once you become a guest, you are positioned as the resident fitness expert. So, if you can't have your own show, be a guest on someone else's.

Rebates/Refunds

This is an excellent way to get people to do business with you. The one thing people love next to getting something for nothing is getting money back. Just look at how many people shop with coupons and send in for rebate offers. If you use a rebate/refund program in your fitness business, make certain you have a way to collect the customer's name, address and telephone number for your mailing list. Also, make sure that everyone on your staff is aware of the program, how it works, and what to expect when a rebate or refund is requested. Your staff must also have the authority to make exceptions on the spot without having to get other approvals. This can occur if the redemption date has expired or the rebate program has changed for an unknown reason.

One rebate program that has been used successfully in several clubs, and also in employee fitness programs, is to return a portion of the membership fee to the member if he or she attends the facility a certain percentage of time within a given time period. This type of program has many beneficial effects. It motivates members to continue to work out because they know they will receive money back. Then, they tell their friends that if you join this club and work out a certain number of times, you get a rebate. This builds a tremendous referral network for you.

The program benefits you because you get a constant influx of new members through the referral system. You are also collecting names for a valuable mailing list to support your other marketing efforts.

Recall/Reactivation Programs

These are usually mail or telephone programs that try to get former members to rejoin the facility or to return to health promotion programs. Fitness professionals would do well to establish recall and reactivation programs, especially as they go through their past membership and attendance records.

A recall or reactivation program has to show concern for the member/customer. The program cannot be a blatant request or demand that they come back to do business with you. Just think about what would attract you to your facility again and then communicate that friendly message to your former customers.

Reception Room

If you have a waiting room in your office, or anywhere in the facility, change the signs and the thinking of the staff to call it a reception room. People hate to wait, but they enjoy being received.

Reception Room Resume

This works well for physicians, attorneys, and accountants, and it will work equally well for a fitness professional. Type up your resume on two sides of a page, laminate it and leave it in the reception room or the lobby for customers (members) to read. Do the same for your fitness staff, and other professionals. In fact, you may want to hang each person's picture next to their resume or have their pictures printed on the resumes and then hang them on the walls. Customers and members will be very impressed, plus they will enjoy learning about the person they are doing business with. The key to a successful reception room/ lobby resume is to keep it informative without seeming like you are patting yourself on the back too much.

Referrals

Every fitness business needs them, but not enough businesses ask for them. Referrals are the heart of every successful fitness business, or any business, for that matter. In fact, there are many businesses in all fields that work strictly on a referral basis.

The first way to build a referral business is to establish a referral network. You refer business to other people, and then these people refer business to you. You make certain they reciprocate and refer back to you by asking them to do so. Just like with your new business request letters, you should describe a potential customer to your referral source. You can't get the business if you do not ask for the business.

Another way to increase referrals is to establish a tiered referral reward system. This rewards current customers as they continue to refer new customers into the facility. The more customers referred in, the greater (in perceived value) the reward. The tiered referral reward system acts as an incentive to continue to do business with you as well as to refer new customers.

Reminders

Simply call, write or send a card to someone to remind them they have an appointment with you. They will appreciate the personal touch and the extra effort on your part.

Reprints

Duplicate any articles that you publish, that are written about you, or that mention your company or your name. Also, reproduce any ads or advertorials you may use. Send these to prospective and current customers to give them an idea of your fitness business, how it operates, and how well it serves people. You should also place these reprints in your media kit.

If you can afford to, take the original of these items to a printer and have them reproduced professionally. They will look better than a photocopy. Or, if the publication provides you with or sells reprints, take theirs because they all will look like an original.

Response Compression

This is another technique that enables you to contact people more often. The high frequency of contact leads to familiarity with your fitness facility, product or service and can lead to increased business. An example of response compression would be if you sent out a mailing to a certain zip code, then three days later you called everyone who received the mailing to invite them to your facility, and five days later you sent another mailing followed by another telephone call, all with a similar sales message. Response compression has been shown to increase response rates to a sales offer by up to five times.

Sales Letters

Sales letters are simply letters to customers, members and prospects announcing a sale on your current membership prices, fitness products, programs and services or the introduction of a new product or service. These letters often contain a discount or value coupon as a call to action for the customer to come in and buy now. The coupons are also dated to create the sense of urgency, especially since you are using the sales letter to create a short-term increase in revenues. Sales letters are effective as marketing tools because they are personalized and cost you just a postage stamp.

Sales Promotions

Sales promotions vary in the type of promotion and the cost to you. The simplest promotion is a discount coupon, such as 25% off a one-year membership or a seminar series, while a more complex promotion is an on-going contest or sweepstakes. The purpose of any sales promotion is to draw attention to your fitness business and to get people involved in the purchase process.

Sales promotions can be done on an individual basis or as a cooperative effort between two or more businesses. In either case, there is usually some discount offer provided to the public. A very inexpensive promotion, and one that generates a great deal of publicity along with customer traffic, is to provide a product, program or service at a slight discount if the customer comes in to the center and makes a donation to a cause. This donation can be a can of food to feed the hungry people in your city. The media will pick up on your efforts and give you a great deal of free coverage for your charitable efforts.

Another inexpensive and highly effective sales promotion is to donate a portion of your proceeds, class fees or guest fees, on a given day to a charity or your local school system. Again, the media loves this type of event. With this promotion, you may not even need to discount your fitness products or services.

The key to effective sales promotions is to plan them wisely, attend to the details, and inform the media of your efforts. Then, you get more than twice the bang for your buck.

Sampling

Sampling is giving away free items or tries of your fitness product or service. You offer prospects samples of your exercise classes for free, a free one week membership, or a free cholesterol screening. These are all effective uses of sampling to get people to do business with you.

Sampling is often used when a fitness company is trying to break into a market, introduce a new product or service, or lure customers from a competitor. People are very willing to take a free sample of something, and if your sample interests them enough, they will possibly switch to what you are selling (health and fitness programs and services). Basically, you are giving something away now to get customers/members to repurchase at a later date.

Searchlight

A giant searchlight is a fabulous attention getter for your fitness center or business if you remain open at night, or you are having a grand opening in the evening. The searchlight lights up the sky and draws people to its source, which is your business location. The rental cost is minimal and the number of people it attracts is maximal. Your responsibility is to sell them once they come into the club.

Seminars, Speeches and Workshops

Any of these three are superb ways to become known in the community, to develop credibility as an expert on the subjects of health and fitness, and to become respected for your contribution to the community. You have several options with seminars, speeches and workshops. If you decide to put on your own seminar or workshop, remember this: it can become very costly because of the printing and mailing costs associated with flyers, brochures and advertising. However, if you have a topic that you know will attract enough people, such as effortless weight loss, (ha, ha) then by all means, conduct the seminar. Only you can decide if you should charge a fee, and what that fee should be, for the seminar.

You can also gain your speaking reputation by contacting professional, civic and social organizations and offering to speak to their membership. The more speeches you give, the more people you will meet. This can translate into more customers for your fitness business, both facility members and corporate clients. Of course, you must decide whether or not you will charge for your speeches. If you are just starting out, give these speeches for free so that you will have an opportunity to get on the programs. Then, as people from one group begin to recommend you to other groups, you can consider charging for your presentation.

Serial Appointments

This works for physicians, accountants, lawyers, tailors, and anyone else who has to meet a customer on several occasions. It will also work if you provide personal training services, weight loss or other types of counseling, new member orientations and workout schedules, and any other service that requires several appointments. Scheduling serial appointments at the time of the initial meeting "commits" the customer to continuing to do business with you. When you combine this with confirmation calls, cards or letters, or your recall program, you have a very effective marketing and customer service tool to keep customers coming back to you.

Share Office Space

This simple idea allows you to save money, market yourself to a potential referral source along with that person's customers, and meet other people in similar situations who will be glad to refer to you. Sharing office space, as they do in executive suites, has become popular for these reasons. Think of all the contacts you can make within a building that allows businesses to share office space.

You may want to have your corporate offices outside the club in a separate office building. Or, you may want to rent space within your facility to another health professional, such as a dietician. Then, you can cross refer to each other. Or, if you are a fitness consultant, you may want to share space with another healthcare or medical professional in a location with other potential clients.

Shop Your Competitors

Most businesses and fitness directors are aware of the need to know what their competitors are doing, but few actually shop them. Shopping your competitors involves actually going to their club, perhaps even spending money there to see how they price their memberships, products and services. Check out how they treat their customers, collect brochures, advertisements and other information about their business, and then identify their weaknesses so you can capitalize on them. The more you know about your competition in your primary service area, the more effective you will be in the fitness marketplace.

Signage

Many fitness businesses fail because nobody knew where they were located or what they were offering. If you have an office or a store front where you conduct your fitness business, make sure the signage is visible from the street, is on the building, on your windows, and anywhere else you are allowed to place a sign. You may even hang a banner across the building or from poles in your parking lot. The goal is to have better than adequate signage that can be read from the street and that directs people to your business. When you use outdoor signs, be sure to check with the building manager and city manager for any codes the building or city may have regarding the use and size of signs.

Signs can also help you if your location is less than ideal. Well designed and informative streetside signs can direct people to your office or facility, even if you are not on a main road. Some clubs have chosen to be off the main road to save on overhead, and they use signs as directional devices.

Also, you must consider the signage within your facility. Make them easy to read, accurate, pleasant to look at, and locate them in appropriate places. Members, guests and customers will truly appreciate your use of good signage.

Shows

Television, radio and news shows are an excellent outlet for your fitness marketing efforts. Both television and radio talk shows enjoy having local professionals and business people as guests. Find out who the producer is of such a show, contact him or her and offer to be a guest. You will probably have to send some information or go down to the station in person to meet the producer, but this effort is well worthwhile considering the exposure you may be getting.

If they have used other fitness professionals on their shows, provide them with a new angle or approach. Create a new way to work out faster and more effectively with less soreness, develop a home exercise program that promotes muscle gain with fat loss and weight loss, or debunk some favorite myths about health and fitness. You get the idea. You must be creative in your approaches to topics when you seek to be a guest on a show.

Call up your local news stations and offer to be a resource for them on health and fitness topics. If they use you on a newscast, you will be perceived as an expert by the viewing public and your credibility will skyrocket. Your business should also improve as a result of your appearance.

Specialty Advertising and Promotions

Specialty advertising and promotions are the inexpensive, little gifts and knick-knacks that your fitness company gives away to customers, members and prospects. These novelty items are printed or engraved with the company name, logo and message. Some specialty advertising items include calendars, keychains, watches, drinking mugs, pens, pads, plastic and duffle bags, gym bags, gym shorts, socks, writing pads, glassware, address books, caps, clocks, tee shirts, and many other things. The purpose of using specialty advertising is to keep your message in front of customers and prospects "all year long" when you cannot be there in person.

Sponsorships

Sponsor a team or an event in your community, such as a little league, softball, soccer, football or basketball team, a race or other sporting event, a special community activity, a fundraiser for a charity, an aerobics contest or marathon, or some other event. Your sponsorship is acknowledged on all the printed material associated with the event or league, on the uniforms if it is a team sponsorship, in the group newsletters, and often times, in the local media. You should also inform the press about your sponsorship as a community contribution to increase your chances of publicity.

Sponsorships generate on-going marketing and advertising for your business as well as an enormous amount of good will. People will see your name on a continuous basis, and familiarity breeds credibility and security. They will want to do business with you. And, think of the positive perceptual link between your being a fitness business and sponsoring a health or related fitness event. The public and the media will love it.

Stamps (Postage)

There are two simple rules of thumb that you should use if you want to get a business envelope opened. The first is always use first class postage. The second is consider using more stamps to equal the required amount of first class postage. For example, a single business letter in 1992 requires $.29 postage. Instead of one stamp, put on five 5 cent stamps and four 1 cent stamps. The person who receives your letter may become intrigued by the number of stamps and open your letter just to see who it is from.

You can also consider using special stamps, such as commemorative or scenic stamps. These also will arouse interest on a business letter and get the envelope opened.

Staff Training *(see In-Service Training, also)*

Ongoing training for your staff is probably the most effective marketing tool you can use. A knowledgeable staff can serve customers better, sell more memberships, fitness products or services, and create an atmosphere in which people like to exercise. Fitness companies, and other business, are finally realizing that it is less expensive and more effective to invest in training their current staff to develop new and improved skills than it is to constantly recruit new staff and train them to acceptable performance standards.

Staff training also motivates employees to stay with your fitness company, and customers like the stability of seeing the same faces every time they come in to work out or attend a class. Also, a well trained staff makes your job as a fitness director that much easier.

Stuffers

Make up a flyer promoting a special class or fitness event, place it in, on or around the gym bag of every customer/member who comes into the facility. Give it to guests who tour the facility or others who just inquire about your fitness services. Contact other businesses and offer to cross promote with them. You will stuff their flyers in your customers'/members' bags if they will stuff yours in their customers' purchases.

The stuffer does not have to be elaborate. It can be a simple coupon or flyer, similar to what you might use in a marriage mailer. The point is to get it into the hands of prospects or customers so that they will be motivated to come back and do business with you.

Tee Shirts (Caps, Gym Bags)

Tee shirts, like baseball caps and gym bags, are an excellent way to have your fitness business and health message seen by the public. You can sell or give the shirts or caps away. Just make sure they promote the message and image you want to project. Tee shirts, caps and gym bags are often viewed as specialty advertising items, but they are mentioned here separately because of their effectiveness in promoting fitness businesses and facilities and the fact that so many businesses neglect to use this message medium.

Tag Lines

Tag lines are simply an extra sentence or two tagged (added) on to your radio, television or print advertisement mentioning a special event, workout, or sale at your club. The tag lines are not a regular part of the promotion and should only be used to announce something that is different and unique from your regular fitness advertising message. These tag lines can also be used to provide a special message to customers, such as saying thank you for their business during a specific period of time. The tag line is virtually a free marketing technique because it is added to already paid-for advertising.

Take One Displays

You see these in supermarkets and department stores. They are flyers or brochures in a display case that says TAKE ONE. The purpose of the display is to attract attention to the flyer or brochure, which then informs customers of a sale or the benefits of coming to your fitness center. Take one displays work very well in high traffic areas, such as malls, where people do not have time to stop for very long, as well as at the checkout counter or cash register or supermarkets or discount stores. They also work well next to impulse items, as customers tend to buy the impulse items and pick up the material from the display at the same time.

The easiest way to get your take one display placed in someone else's business or store is to offer to do a cross promotion with them. Since you are proactively reciprocating, the other businesses will most likely agree to work with you. It becomes a win-win situation for your fitness center and your joint-venture marketing partner.

Telemarketing

The important thing to remember about telemarketing is that it is less expensive to contact a customer by telephone than in person. You can also reach more people in a given time period, allowing you to be more productive in your marketing and sales efforts.

The key to successful telemarketing is a well prepared telemarketer. This means having a person who may not necessarily be another fitness professional but may be someone who can sell on the telephone and who can be trained in your product or service do your telemarketing. They should follow a well-written script and deviate from it only when necessary or after they gain experience. They should keep the conversation natural, and remain courteous to the customer at all times. While some fitness products or services can sell themselves over the telephone, more often than not, it is the skills of the telemarketer that determine the number and dollar amounts of the sales.

One other point must be made about telemarketing. You must track the sales volume it generates to make sure you are getting a good return on your investment in this marketing technique.

Testimonials

When a customer, client or member tells you they are satisfied with the way you conduct your fitness business, or with a purchase they made from you, or with how you helped them get in better shape, ask them to write it in a letter to you. Collect these testimonial letters from as many people as possible. Use them as additional sales and marketing tools. Customers and prospects always like to read about what people just like themselves think of doing business with you. These testimonial letters, and even short quotes, will add credibility to your fitness programs and services.

A good idea is to keep these letters in protective sheets in a three ring binder. This way, all your customers/members can read them without destroying the letter. It also looks very professional to have them in a binder with a cover page.

Toll Booth

This is not so much a true marketing technique as it is a very unique tactic. If you drive to your club and must pay a toll, check your rear view mirror. If the car behind you is expensive, consider paying its toll also. Hand the money and your business card to the booth agent and ask him or her to give the driver of the next car your business card and tell him or her that you paid their toll. When they come through the booth, you should be waiting off to the side. More often than not, drivers of the car behind you will stop to speak with you either out of interest or just sheer curiosity.

Your success ratio may or may not be very high with this tactic, and it may cost you some money, but if one driver becomes a member or a corporate fitness client, this tactic could be worth a try.

Tracking

This is another marketing approach, more so than a technique. Yet, this is definitely one of the most important aspects of your marketing program. Too many fitness directors implement marketing efforts and then fail to track their results. Or, they track them to some degree then do nothing with the results. How can you know if your fitness marketing efforts are effective and successful if you do not track them?

Always ask customers and new members where they heard about you, or who referred them to you. All flyers and coupons should have a code on them so you can track them when they are returned. Developing effective tracking techniques lets you determine the actual cost of your marketing program and your return on investment. It then allows you to evaluate the program and to make revisions, if necessary.

Trade Shows

These are an excellent way to get your message in front of hundreds of thousands of people for very little cost. Of course, you must figure in the expense of the booth, travel, room and board, and salaries of the people attending the trade show. However, it is worth it if you want to reach large numbers of people committed to buying your fitness programs and services.

You probably have attended many fitness industry trade shows to know what you like and dislike about exhibits. Use that knowledge, then make certain your display is professional and eye catching. Have enough sales literature and business cards to give out. Also, have enough other fitness professionals in your booth to talk to prospects as they come by. Finally, make sure you follow up on every lead from the trade show with a letter, another brochure, and a telephone call. Almost 25% of the leads obtained at trade shows are never followed up on. That is just too much potential business to let go to waste.

Unique Sales Proposition (USP)

Every fitness business needs one, but only a few actually determine what their unique sales proposition is. The USP differentiates your marketing and sales message from your competitors'. Your USP must be made in conjunction with your Unique Marketing Position (UMP). This is the statement that positions you in the minds of your consumers. The USP and the UMP combined often determine how successful your business will be.

To determine your USP, ask yourself what it is you are really selling, and see if that is what customers are really buying. If there is a match, write it down. If there is not a match, look at your fitness product, program or service from the customer's viewpoint. Then, write your USP from that perspective.

Upselling

Upselling is an effective marketing technique that requires your staff to sell the customer/member what he or she wants, then sell them more of the same or add another product or service to the sale. It is very closely related to cross-selling, which involves selling customers related products or services simultaneously.

When you upsell someone, you are still trying to satisfy their needs, wants and expectations. You are just adding more value to the sale, and of course, a higher price. It's like buying a club membership and then purchasing a series of health promotion screenings on top of the membership. "Bait and Switch" advertising however is illegal and must be avoided.

Value Added Service

Providing value added service is a superb way to differentiate your business from competitors. This means you will give customers more for their money. You may extend the three day cooling off period to five days when someone joins your club, or you may deliver a corporate program to a location that is some distance from your facility without charging for travel, or just go out of your way to give your customers something extra. You are giving added value (and service) to the purchase they are making. Value added service all but guarantees they will purchase from you again and also refer their family and friends to you. It costs you nothing and gains you a great deal.

Vendor Support Programs

These types of programs are often used with special events, such as a facility grand opening or open house. You contact your vendors or suppliers, inform them of what you are doing, and ask them to make a financial contribution to the event. In return, you will give them media exposure in your local area through the newspaper, radio and television ads you will use to promote the event.

Vendors are often quite happy to participate in these programs. The programs are similar to co-op marketing programs, and vendors usually have millions of dollars available every year in support and co-op programs that go unused. The reason is that nobody asks the vendors for these funds.

Volunteer

Volunteer for a community service organization, committee or charity. Get out and be seen. Become a member of a service organization, sit on their committees or boards, help out with their events. Work for a charity. Customers view fitness professionals and companies whose people volunteer in a very favorable light. They often choose to join your club or participate in your programs just because of your civic mindedness.

It is true being a volunteer will take some of your time, but it is time well invested. The contacts you will make and the public image you will create are invaluable. Plus, you will definitely feel good about helping others.

Volunteers

Don't only be a volunteer, use volunteers. Many people, especially retirees, are eager to volunteer to help a business help people, especially a fitness center. You probably already have special programs just for seniors. Expand your penetration into this market by hiring seniors as employees and allowing others to volunteer at your facility. You can use volunteers to act as hosts or hostesses, guides, customer service people, or in any capacity you can think of. Not only does this help your business, it also creates a favorable image to customers and the general public.

Another form of volunteerism is student interns from the local high schools and colleges. The benefits of interns has already been discussed in the section on interns. They bring to your facility a strong desire to learn, motivation to help people, and a background in the fitness field from their schools. Try using volunteers, both retirees and student interns, and you will be pleasantly surprised.

Walk Your Talk

Get down in the trenches with your people and meet your customers/members. Let both your customers and employees know you care about them. Nothing is more effective as a marketing technique than meeting, greeting and speaking with the people who do business with you, work out with you and who run your business for you.

There is nothing you can create or purchase, from public relations to advertising, that can have the effect of personally meeting people. Face to face contact and the personal touch are the most powerful tools any fitness business can have to promote itself. With all the clubs and fitness service providers offering the same high tech equipment and programs, it is very important for you to differentiate yourself by offering high touch. This approach will significantly enhance your word of mouth marketing efforts and your referral network.

Welcome Wagon

This can be an effective tool since new residents are often looking for a place to exercise, lose weight, and even meet new friends. The welcome wagon is a relatively inexpensive program to participate in, and someone else delivers the message for you. Usually, you have to provide a coupon with a discount offer for memberships or classes to the new neighbor.

This approach is worth trying if your offer is intriguing enough to have the person come in to your center. There are both success stories and failures with the welcome wagon, but it can promote you to newcomers fairly inexpensively. You will have to try it yourself and track it to see if it is effective for you.

Word of Mouth

This goes along with walking your talk. Word of mouth, which we discussed earlier in the book, is also known as referrals. Since it can be extremely low cost or no cost, it is often the best way to build a fitness business. When someone refers you to a friend, they have given you instant credibility. The new customer is much more likely to buy from you, or join your club, than if they had to come in to see you on their own. Then, if you satisfy the new customer, that person will also refer others to you. Your entire business can be built on word of mouth marketing.

In a similar vein, word of mouth marketing can hurt your fitness business. Just think of a club or business that does not deliver on its promises or does not sell what it advertises. It can take them up to 10 years to recover from poor word of mouth. That is why word of mouth, combined with a fitness director walking the talk, are the most powerful marketing techniques available.

Writing

Write and publish articles, books or monographs. If you cannot find someone to publish these for you, publish them yourself. A published book or booklet on fitness gives you instant credibility as an expert, and everyone likes to do business with an expert. The same is true for articles and monographs. People believe whatever they read in print. It must be fact, otherwise why would it be printed? And if you wrote the facts, you must be the expert. Therefore, do everything you can to get something published. The effort will be very worthwhile.

Yellow Pages

Your Yellow Pages representative will tell you that every business, especially fitness centers and service providers, needs to be listed, and that a display ad is better than a line ad, and that a large ad is better than a small ad, and that red is better than black. The only business that these things are better for is the Yellow Pages provider.

If you are going to use the Yellow Pages as a marketing vehicle, consider the neighborhood directories as well as the regional directory. You must also consider the type of ad you will place. Unique listings can be more effective than large or colorful listings. For example, create your own category, then you will have no competition.

If you can afford it, you may want to consider multiple line listings in several categories. There is an easy way to determine where you should place your listings. Just ask your customers where they would look for you if they were to use the Yellow Pages. Then place the listings in those categories they recommended most often. Of course, place at least a line listing in the section on health clubs and gyms.

One other point about Yellow Pages. They are effective, when used properly. That means having a professional create your ad so that it is in concert with your entire marketing campaign. It also means having the ad sell your fitness business and services, not just giving your name and telephone number in the ad. On the other side of the coin, the Yellow Pages can be a big, ineffective investment. Here again, you must track the business it brings in. If you are paying for a large ad and you are not getting at least a 10:1 return on the investment for that ad, perhaps you should reconsider this as a marketing tool.

A Final Word to the Successful Fitness Director

Plan to market your fitness business in the least expensive, most effective manner possible. It is marketing that drives a fitness business, nothing else. All the promotional techniques, such as advertising, public relations, customer service, selling, sales promotions, etc., are just sub-categories of marketing.

Most fitness businesses do not have the budgets of the mega-corporations and mega-chains, yet they can be just as effective in their marketing efforts if they use these implementation techniques. It is definitely possible for a small club or company to compete with a large one on equal ground using many of these low cost, no cost marketing techniques.

Be patient with your marketing program. Allow it enough time to work. Evaluate the program carefully and honestly and make changes when and where they are necessary. Although these techniques are simple and inexpensive, you should try them and see how much they improve your fitness business. You will be pleasantly surprised. Good luck.

Appendix A
Marketing Action Pack

Here, in a nutshell, are the forms, charts and tables I have used successfully over the years to help companies, consultants, clubs, wellness centers, and all types of businesses develop effective and profitable marketing programs. All you have to do is answer the questions, fill in the charts, and gather the information that is requested. Also, feel free to adapt any of the material to suit your needs.

Market Business Analysis

What is the mission/nature of the business?

What corporate image does the business have?

What are the products/programs/services the business offers?

Who are the customers and where are they located?

What are their primary needs and desired benefits?

What unique positioning does the business hold?

Who are the competitors and what is their market share?

What are the most effective promotional tactics?

When and how will the products/programs/services be distributed?

What are the resource requirements for the business?

Target Market Attractiveness Rating Scale

CRITERIA	ATTRACTIVENESS				
	LOW			HIGH	
Market Size	1	2	3	4	5
Market Growth Potential	1	2	3	4	5
Client Accessibility	1	2	3	4	5
User Potential	1	2	3	4	5
Payment Capabilities	1	2	3	4	5
Entry/Exit Potential	1	2	3	4	5
Competition	1	2	3	4	5
Referral Potential	1	2	3	4	5
Service/Program Awareness/Recognition	1	2	3	4	5
Service/Program Need	1	2	3	4	5

SWOT Analysis

STRENGTHS	WEAKNESSES

OPPORTUNITIES	THREATS

Competitor Analysis: Marketing Mix

COMPETITOR'S NAME: _____ DATE: _____

PRODUCT/PROGRAM/SERVICE NAME:
Production Costs:
Supplier Relations:

PRICING STRATEGY:
Leader/Follower:
Price Position:

PLACE/DISTRIBUTION CHANNELS:
Primary:
Secondary:
Distributor Relations:
System Advantages/Disadvantages:

PROMOTION:
Types:
Quality/Effectiveness:

POSITIONING:
Target Market/Niche/Segmentation:
Unique Features/Benefits/Attributes/Uses:

SERVICE POLICY:
Product/Program/Service Support:
Customer Support:

Competitors' Comparative Characteristics

CHARACTERISTIC	YOUR COMPANY	COMPETITOR A	COMPETITOR B	COMPETITOR C
1. Geographic Boundaries				
2. Target Markets				
3. Market Segmentation Procedures				
4. Marketing Strategies and Tactics				
5. Marketing Assumptions				
6. Marketing Mix				
7. Program/Products/ Services Offered				
8. Operating Costs/ Assumptions				
9. Market Share				
10. Marketplace Entry/Exit, Stage of Life Cycle				

Product/Service Evaluation

MISSION STATEMENT/RATIONALE:

GOALS AND OBJECTIVES:

COMPANY STRENGTHS AND WEAKNESSES:

COMPETITOR STRENGTHS AND WEAKNESSES:

TARGET MARKET/UNIQUE POSITIONING:

COSTS/RESOURCES REQUIRED:

SERVICE AREA:

DISTRIBUTION METHODS:

CUSTOMER SERVICE PROGRAM:

EVALUATION TECHNIQUES:

TIME REQUIREMENTS:

CRITICAL ISSUES:

Target Market Characteristics

Characteristic	PRIMARY	SECONDARY
Location	_____	_____
Age	_____	_____
Gender	_____	_____
Income	_____	_____
Education	_____	_____
Occupation	_____	_____
Marital Status	_____	_____
Family Size	_____	_____
Family Life Cycle	_____	_____
Buying Influences	_____	_____
Benefits Sought	_____	_____
User Status	_____	_____
Usage Rates	_____	_____
Loyalty Status	_____	_____
Attitudes	_____	_____
Readiness State	_____	_____
Race/Religion/Nationality	_____	_____
Lifestyle	_____	_____
Social Class	_____	_____
Personality	_____	_____

Goals and Strategies For
The Marketing Mix

What does the company want to achieve this year?

_____

_____

_____

How much money do we want to make? What is our desired profit margin?

_____

Where is the industry in the Product Life Cycle (introductory, growth, maturity, declining) and what strategies are necessary to compete in this phase? _____

_____

_____

Who is our target market and what is our unique position in their minds?

_____

_____

What is our time frame for achieving our business and financial goals?

_____

What resources do we have to implement the necessary tactics to achieve the strategies we develop in the marketing mix? _____

_____

Are there any specific legal ramifications or requirements related to our product or service? _____

_____

Do we have the required licenses, patents, trademarks and registrations for our product or service? _____

_____

Does our product or service infringe on any currently trademarked or registered product or service? If so, how will we overcome this obstacle?

_____

_____

Developing The Marketing Mix

1. Target market selection/market segmentation characteristics:

2. Products/programs/services offered:
    Name: _____

    Features   **Benefits**   **Need Satisfaction**

3. Distribution channels (accessibility and availability):

4. Price (includes discounts, incentive and payment terms):

5. Promotion:
    A. Types of communications:

    B. Techniques:
        1.   Advertising
        2.   Publicity
        3.   Public relations
        4.   Business publications: brochures, flyers
        5.   Direct mail
        6.   Personal selling
        7.   Telemarketing
        8.   Networking
        9.   Speeches
        10. Community service

Follow the form above to develop your own marketing mix.

Fill in one sheet for each product or service you offer. Every product or service, or every different market you serve, should have its own marketing mix.

Creative Development Plan

Project: Date:

Goal/Strategy:

Primary Tactics:

_____

1.   What is the key problem or opportunity?

2.   What is the primary marketing objective to be achieved?

3.   What results are expected from this marketing program?

4.   Who are our target customers and competitors?

5.   What benefits do we offer our customers?

6.   What is our unique positioning or niche?

7.   What promotional tactics will be used?

8.   How will the effectiveness of the program be measured?

9.   What constraints (budget, media, staff, etc.) exist for this program?

10.   What other critical issues must be considered?

Appendix B

The Ten Greatest Fitness Marketing Techniques

Someone said there was a recession going on, but if you were marketing your fitness business properly, you would never feel its effects. In fact, you probably would be making a substantial profit right now.

Many fitness businesses are scrambling trying to get new members or participants and trying to outdo their competition in one way or another. Some are spending lavish amounts of money on advertising, promotions, or offering deep discounts to keep their cash flowing. You will never have to do this if you develop and implement a marketing plan that includes one, or more or all of the following ten greatest fitness marketing techniques of all time.

Ten Marketing Techniques to Make Your Fitness Business More Profitable

1. *Unique Selling Proposition (USP) and Unique Marketing Position (UMP)*
   Most businesses do not have either of these important factors. Your USP is exactly why people should purchase your fitness products or services. It is what differentiates you from the competition and what makes your fitness business unique.

   Your UMP is the marketing position you hold in their minds, such as being the friendliest fitness center or program provider in town, or the most service-oriented club, or the lowest price provider. Having both a USP and UMP will place you significantly ahead of your competition and force them to play catch-up.

2. *Recall and Reactivation Programs*
   These programs involve contacting members or customers who have not been in to see you for some time, say six months or a year. You should call or write them to find out how they are doing and invite them in for a special program, sale or trial membership. Remember that your former customers are your gold mine. Sometimes, they just have to be reminded about your products or services, what you do for them and how well you do it. It is much easier to get them to come back to see you than to try to find new customers, participants or members. Once you have them back, it is essential that you convert them to full time program participants.

3. *Customer Recognition and Reward Programs*
   Your fitness business needs referrals to survive. Therefore, you should develop a referral reward program for your customers and members. Put their names up on a "Thank You" bulletin board in the club or office. Send cards and letters thanking them. Then, as they continue to refer, send them gifts of progressively increasing values. This tiered reward program shows your referral sources you care about them and you appreciate the effort they are making on your behalf. This is also known as a frequent referrers program. You can modify this to be a frequent buyer program by giving customers who buy from you often greater discounts or free products or services.

Also, customers appreciate fitness directors and business owners who appreciate them. Send your customers holiday and birthday cards, congratulatory letters, and thank you cards or letters when they refer new customers to you. Show them you care about them personally, and they will return the favor by referring new customers to you, by purchasing more from you, and by remaining loyal to you.

4. **Letter of News**
Newsletters help you keep in touch with your customers and members as well as keep them informed. However, these people probably receive quite a few newsletters. In order to make your information stand out from the crowd, and definitely keep your name in front of the customers, you should send a letter of news. This is simply a personal letter to the customer or member that contains all the information that would have normally been in the newsletter, but now it has been personalized. People will read personal letters much faster and more completely than they will a newsletter.

5. **Charity Tie-Ins and Community Service**
Get involved with a local charity or sponsor a community event or sports team. Your civic-mindedness will definitely be rewarded. Customers like to do business with companies, clubs and programs that give something back to the community. Also, remember to publicize your involvement.

6. **Public Identity**
The identity you create for yourself and your business will follow you wherever you go. Write articles, give speeches, send out press releases on newsworthy events related to your business. Be available to customers, be visible to the community, and always speak to the media if they call. Remember that your public image is only the perception people have of you at a given moment in time, but your public identity is the physical, mental and emotional embodiment of that image all the time. It is who and what you and your business are.

7. **Direct Response Advertising**
Too many clubs and fitness businesses advertise in print, on radio and television and place what is called institutional or tombstone ads. These are technical or information giving ads that do nothing to motivate the customer to call or come into the facility. Your ads, and this includes your Yellow Pages ad, must be a sales piece that motivates the customer to call, write or come into your facility. You must also track the effectiveness of each ad you place to make certain you are getting a good return for your advertising dollar. ALL ADVERTISING MUST BE DIRECT RESPONSE.

8. **Sampling, Discounts and Coupons**
Businesses give away free samples of products or services all the time. They also offer discounts and coupons to motivate people to try their product or service. This is especially true when they are offering something new to customers and they want to see how customers will respond. You should always consider doing this, as long as it is cost effective. The return on this investment, such as customers making subsequent purchases, must be sufficient to support a sampling program.

9. ***Service Guarantees, Risk Reversals and Easily Accessible, User Friendly Customer Service Systems***

Whatever type of fitness program or service you provide, give the people a guarantee. Make it full money back and unconditional. People will appreciate your confidence in your product or service plus they will feel very comfortable with you because you are taking all the risk. Most people will not take advantage of your service guarantees. They will, however, continue to do business with you as long as you provide them value for their money.

Also, make your customer service systems easy to use. The systems must be more than complaint handling. They must be designed to ensure customer and member satisfaction at all times. Employees must be trained and empowered to take responsibility and make decisions that will ultimately help and satisfy the customer. Once customers are satisfied, you must go beyond customer service to guarantee customer loyalty, future purchases and an on-going referral system.

10. ***Everybody Sells***

This is a mental attitude you must impart to your entire staff. Everybody markets, everybody sells. Now, sales must be combined with service and the knowledge of how to communicate with people (developing rapport and interpersonal style). Successful sales professionals know how to identify their customers' needs, expectations, wants and satisfiers. These sales professionals also market their products or services so that the "job" of selling becomes easier. Finally, these sales professionals listen more than they speak, negotiate with customers to achieve a beneficial win-win solution for both parties, and service their customers to the best of their abilities and beyond their customers' expectations.

In short, successful fitness businesses market and sell their products and services in ways that develop rapport, trust and long term relationships with their customers. Achieving these outcomes is the only way anyone can retain customers and keep them for life.

These are the ten greatest fitness marketing techniques of all time. Fitness businesses across the country, from personal trainers to large clubs, corporate and hospital fitness centers, have been taught to use these tools as part of their marketing programs. Their success has been unparalleled. Use one, a combination, or preferably, all ten and you will realize tremendous success in your fitness business.

Appendix C

10 Greatest Customer/Member Service and Retention Tips of All Time*

1. ### *Unique Service Philosophy (USP)*
   Fitness businesses need a unique service philosophy or mission statement. This USP should compliment their overall business mission statement. The Unique Service Philosophy should describe exactly how customer/members will be treated when they purchase memberships, products, programs and services from you. The USP should also describe your preferred outcomes for every service encounter.

2. ### *Customer/Member Feedback*
   Get customer/member feedback any way you can. Set up customer/member councils, focus groups, hand out surveys in your facility, mail out surveys, conduct personal interviews, and beg your customers/members for feedback. The more you involve customer/members with your business, the more they will tell you how to improve it to satisfy them. Listen, evaluate the information, and then act on the suggestions.

3. ### *Service and Retention Programs*
   Use your customer/member service system and your customer/member retention program as a powerful marketing tool. Call your customer/members, send them thank you and holiday cards, mail them newsletters. Do anything and everything you can to keep them informed about your fitness business and how important they are to your success. The more your name is in front of them, the greater the probability they will continue to do business with you.

4. ### *Close the Gap*
   Quite often, a gap exists between what customer/members expect from a fitness business and what they actually receive. There is also a gap between what the fitness business thinks customer/members want and what the customer/members actually want. You must constantly work to close these gaps so your perceptions of situations are in line with those of your customer/members.

5. ### *Meet and Exceed Expectations*
   Customer/members have certain expectations they bring to every business situation. You must meet these expectations just to satisfy the customer/member. You must exceed these expectations to ensure their long term loyalty, membership and referral potential. Exceeding expectations is the key to retention and re-purchase.

6. *Customer/Member Reward Programs*

What gets rewarded gets done. Any type of reward program aimed at the customer/ member, such as frequent buyer or referral programs, will motivate the customer/ member to continue purchasing from you. Rewards make the customer/member feel special, and they will keep coming back to the source of that special feeling. (You should also do this for your employees.)

7. *Public Identity*

The identity you create for your business must match the perceived identity customer/ members have of themselves. This is just one factor they use in deciding to join your facility or participate in your programs. The image and identity you create in the community, backed up by your actions, influences when and how long customers/ members do business with you.

8. *Community Service*

Community service, charity tie-ins and environmental issues have a large influence on customer/member expectations for doing business with a fitness company. Make sure your customer/members know of your efforts in these areas. This will help them feel good about doing business with you.

9. *Easily Accessible, User Friendly Service Systems*

Make it extremely easy for customer/members to get service from you. When they need something from you, have it for them. This includes new fitness products or programs, returns, refunds, resolving complaints, or anything else they need. Keep your rules, regulations, policies and procedures flexible. They should only be guidelines, not laws.

10. *Train and Empower Your Employees*

Quality employees provide quality service. Education, degrees and certification are important, but they are not enough. Your employees must be trained. Train your employees in their job tasks and in providing superior customer/member service. Then, give your employees the authority to make decisions to satisfy the customer/ member, even if it goes against company policy. Support your employees in all their decisions to satisfy and keep the customer/member. After all, without customer/ members, there is no business.

* Any overlap with or repetition of one or several of the 10 Greatest Fitness Marketing Techniques of All Time is purely intentional.

Seven Steps To Successful
Customer/Member Retention

1. Have a clear customer service mission, vision and philosophy. Communicate this to your employees, then train and empower them to carry out your service mission to your external customers.

2. Provide customers with quality fitness products, programs, services and care.

3. Listen closely to your customers, employees and members. Then act on their suggestions.

4. Pay attention to your own intuition when serving customers, and have your employees pay attention to their own intuitions. Then, turn your intuitions into action.

5. Treat your customers and members with respect, trust, fairness, honesty and integrity. Make them feel important.

6. Communicate with your customers regularly, including current customers, former customers and your competitor's customers.

7. Expand your fitness product, program and service offerings carefully, ensuring you can continue to provide quality customer service while you grow.

Barriers To Effective
Customer Service And Retention

1.   Poor attitudes on the part of the fitness company and its employees towards the customers.

2.   The fitness director's employees' or company's inability to fully understand the customer's current and long-term needs, wants and expectations.

3.   The fitness company does not possess the resources to service the customer properly.

4.   Poor organization of the customer service program.

5.   Rigid and inflexible policies and procedures regarding customer service.

6.   Employees do not listen or respond to customers.

7.   Employees do not provide customers or members with individualized attention.

8.   The fitness company and its employees do not respond to customer feedback, recommendations and suggestions.

9.   Employees and the company project a poor image, such as being out of shape, poorly dressed, or having a dirty facility.

10. Employees have too much to do with their jobs and not enough time to service the customers/members or implement the retention programs.

10 Commandments of Superior Customer/Member Service and Retention

1. The customer/member is the most important person in the company.

2. The customer/member is not dependent on you or your staff. Rather, you are all dependent upon the customer/member. You work for the customer/member. You work for the customer/member.

3. The customer/member is not an interruption of your work. The customer/member is the purpose of your work.

4. The customer/member does you a favor by visiting or calling or joining your facility. You are not doing the customer/member a favor by serving them.

5. The customer/member is as much a part of your fitness business as anything else, including inventory, employees and your facility. If you sold the fitness business, the customer/members would go with it.

6. The customer/member is not a cold statistic. The customer/member is a person with feelings and emotions, just like you. Treat the customer/member better than you would want to be treated.

7. The customer/member is not someone to argue with or to match wits with. You and your business will be the only losers.

8. It is your job to satisfy the needs, wants and expectations of your customer/members, and whenever possible, resolve their fears and complaints.

9. The customer/member deserves the most attentive, courteous and professional treatment you and your staff can provide.

10. The customer/member is the lifeblood of your fitness business. Always remember that without customer/members, you would not have a fitness business.

10 Tips For Long Term
Customer/Member Retention

1. Call each customer/member by name. Ask them if they prefer their first name only, or to be addressed as Mr., Mrs., or Ms.

2. Listen to what each customer/member has to say. Pay close and careful attention and let them know you are paying attention to them.

3. Be concerned about each customer/member as an individual. If you treat each one as a member of your family, the favor will be rewarded tenfold.

4. Be courteous, polite and respectful to each customer/member.

5. Be responsive to the individual needs of each customer/member. Personalize the attention you provide to them.

6. Know their personal buying history and motivations. Know the best and most conductive way to sell them additional programs and services. Never make them feel uncomfortable in your facility.

7. Take sufficient time with each customer/member. Make them feel they are the most important person in the world at this particular time.

8. Involve customer/members in your fitness business. Ask for their advice and suggestions, then act upon them.

9. Make customer/members feel important. Pay them honest compliments. Acknowledge their achievements and those of their family members.

10. Listen first to understand the customer/member. Then, speak so they can understand you.

Customer/Member's Bill of Rights

The customer/member has a right to the following:

1. Professional, courteous and prompt service in all areas of the fitness center or any of its programs.

2. Your full and undivided attention each time the customer/member chooses to do business with you or speak to you.

3. Quality fitness products, programs and services.

4. Fulfillment of needs in a manner consistent with reasonable service expectations, such as having equipment available to exercise on even during peak hours and having instructors show up on time to teach classes.

5. Competent, knowledgeable and well-trained staff. If your staff has degrees and certifications, and they should, let your customer/members know this.

6. Attention to every detail every time they access your customer/member service system. Remember that it is the minor details that make the major difference in your success.

7. The benefits of all of your resources, teamwork and networks to provide superior and long-term service, even if they let their membership lapse or stop attending classes.

8. Open channels of communication to provide feedback and voice complaints or compliments, without you or your staff becoming defensive or argumentative.

9. A fair and reasonable price for the fitness memberships, products, programs or services they are purchasing.

10. Appreciation on the part of you and your staff for the business already given and the business that will be given in the future, including referrals to friends and family.

A Final Thought

Always remember that your employees are your first line of customers. These internal customers must be treated with the same care, respect and importance as your external (buying) customer/members. In order for your employees to provide superior service and work to keep the customer/members, you must provide superior service and working conditions to your employees. Then, you must work harder than ever to keep them.

Index